WHO DO YOU THINK YOU ARE?

WHO DO YOU THINK YOU ARE?

Man or Superman—
The Genetic Controversy

OLIVER GILLIE

SATURDAY REVIEW PRESS / E. P. DUTTON & CO., INC.

NEW YORK

Grateful acknowledgment is made for permission to reprint from the following:

Black Like Me by John Howard Griffin. Copyright © 1962 by John Howard Griffin. Reprinted by permission of Houghton Mifflin Co., Boston, and John Howard Griffin.

The Politics of Experience by R. D. Laing. Copyright © 1967 by R. D. Laing. Reprinted by permission of Penguin Books Ltd., London.

Race, Intelligence and Education by H. J. Eysenck. Copyright © 1971 by H. J. Eysenck. Reprinted by permission of Maurice Temple Smith Ltd., London.

Sexual Politics by Kate Millett. Copyright © 1969, 1970 by Kate Millett. Reprinted by permission of Doubleday & Co., Inc., New York.

Crime and Personality by H. J. Eysenck. Copyright © 1970 by H. J. Eysenck. Reprinted by permission of Routledge and Kegan Paul Ltd., London.

Genetics and Man by C. D. Darlington. Copyright © 1964 by C. D. Darlington. Reprinted by permission of George Allen & Unwin Ltd., London, and Macmillan Publishing Co., Inc., New York.

Crime as Destiny by J. Lange. Copyright 1931 by J. Lange. Reprinted by permission of George Allen & Unwin Ltd., London.

Sex, Gender and Society by Ann Oakley. Copyright © 1972 by Ann Oakley. Reprinted by permission of Maurice Temple Smith Ltd., London, and Harper & Row, New York.

"Educability and Group Differences" by J. N. Thoday. Reprinted by permission of *Nature,* Macmillan Journals Ltd., London.

"Sex, Intersex and the Law," editorial in *The Lancet.* Reprinted by permission of *The Lancet,* London.

Intersexuality by C. N. Armstrong and A. J. Marshall. Reprinted by permission of Academic Press, Inc. Ltd., London.

Published simultaneously in Canada
by Clarke, Irwin & Company
Limited, Toronto and Vancouver

ISBN: 0-8415-0397-4
Library of Congress Cataloging in Publication Data

Gillie, Oliver.
    Who do you think you are?

    Includes bibliographical references and index.
    1. Nature and nurture.   2. Sex.   3. Crime and criminals.
4. Hygiene.   5. Intellect.   I. Title.
BF341.G5 1976   155.2'34   75-25743

For my daughters, Lucinda and Juliet

Acknowledgments

I would like to thank Michael Sissons and Harold Evans—without their encouragement and understanding this book would never have been written. I would like to thank my wife for her forbearance. I would like to thank friends who have commented on the manuscript, particularly Professor Geoffrey Beale. I am also deeply indebted to Caroline Hartnell and Ann La Farge for their expert editing of the manuscript.

Contents

INTELLIGENCE

MAN AND SUPERMAN

WHO DO YOU THINK YOU ARE?

Introduction

Who am I? Why am I who I am? These appear to be simple questions, the kind you asked your parents and expected to have answered and that we ask ourselves, in some form, nearly every day. Like busy parents giving their children convenient answers, we often try to settle the question without considering the facts. Sometimes we answer that we can be whoever we want to be; sometimes we say that our character is predestined. Then comes the next question: Are we born with our own character—have we inherited it—or is it shaped by the events of our lives?

In this book I attempt to show which of our assumptions about ourselves are false and which are true. It is often convenient to believe that we are predestined by heredity for a certain position in life. Widespread acceptance of this idea often makes it a reality and may deprive individuals of the freedom to change themselves on a personal level. But human character is more plastic than we realize: within wide limits, it is molded by the environment. And also within limits, individuals can mold their own character and, in effect, choose the sort of person they wish to become.

Many of us have the potential to change our lives, but relatively few have the time to do so. Perhaps we are trapped within ready-made stereotypes, functioning with less and less enthusiasm in the roles society expects of us: the junior executive who would like to go "back to the land" but cannot escape the office routine; the chicken farmer who wants to be an engineer or musician; the housewife, secretary, or nurse who might run her own business or be a doctor if she just got the chance. Somewhere inside most of us there is someone else—a hundred different people, even—screaming to get out. Before we can change our lives we must believe that change is possible. And when change is difficult, it is easy to believe that human character is fixed by heredity and that change is therefore impossible. Our freewill is limited by our environment and the opportunities it gives us to learn. This restriction of freedom begins in the womb as the baby struggles to grow fully. The bonds are tightened during the first five or ten years of life. The Jesuits say, "Give me a child for seven years and I care not who has him thereafter." These are crucial years, but patterns of behavior can go on changing throughout life; for example, a person's IQ test score may vary from one year to the next.

There is a widespread belief that criminals, madmen, and geniuses—to name only three categories of people—are born rather than made. These notions obtain general support from scientific evidence that appears to show that intelligence, criminality, and, for example, schizophrenia are strongly inherited. However, much of the scientific evidence is based on dubious assumptions that can be traced back to ideological influences.

The views of individual scientists on the nature/nurture issue follow their political beliefs very closely. "Liberal" or "radical" scientists tend to be "environmentalists," and "conservative" scientists tend to be "hereditarians" who believe that heredity is of preeminent importance in deciding character. This is exactly what we might expect when we reflect that it is conservatives who always have the greatest interest in property and titles—that is, the greatest vested interest in nonbiological inheritance. The assumptions of hereditarian science are discreetly clothed in jargon. And after a process of "scientific" laundering, these assumptions surface as apparently authoritative statements such as "intelligence is 80 percent inherited" or "schizophrenia is caused by an inherited biochemical defect."

Prevailing beliefs on the nature/nurture issue inevitably influence the organization of society. Not only do they influence the way we structure our schools, prisons, asylums, and other institutions but they also affect the way we think of ourselves and our fellows. If people believe that their intelligence and general character are largely fixed at birth, they are likely to accept their lot without complaint. A strong belief in the importance of good breeding helps those who are well off to justify their circumstances. The political importance of these themes is shown in the way both the Nazis and the Soviet Communists imprisoned and silenced geneticists.

Much of the scientific work purporting to demonstrate that human intelligence and character are strongly inherited is based on inconclusive data and on arguments containing questionable assumptions. Where human character is concerned, and particularly the character of whole races, science, like the law, should give the benefit of all reasonable doubt to the accused. While I may frequently assert that the hereditarians exhibit a species of dogmatism that smacks more of emotional conviction than of scientific analysis, I must also state that the environmentalists, too, often speak from emotional conviction. I aim to show that science is not neutral, and that the consumer of it must beware when scientists protest, as they so often do, that theirs is the view of experts. As Theodore Roszak has said in his book *The Making of a Counter Culture,* the objective consciousness of scientists is a myth.[1]

The object of this book, then, is to redraw the accepted dividing line between the influences of heredity and environment on our lives and to give much more credit to the environment than the convinced hereditarians have done, particularly when questions of social importance such as racism, sexism, and elitism arise. Science, by favoring hard fact and an abstract approach, is in danger of stripping man of his soft parts, and so presents him to the world as a programmed robot—a slave of his inheritance. The genetic engineer is the mechanic who tinkers with the robot, tuning it for top performance. This popular conception derives from the vision and the ethos of molecular biology, which has presented the possibility of developing a superrace from "cuttings" taken from the tissues of distinguished men and women. This possibility could be realized only if the environment were to count for little.

The concept of the superman and the superrace with inherited strength and virtue has warped our vision of society and of people. The superman cult has infiltrated science with ideas such as the inheritance of genius and intellectual superiority. The antithesis of superman is portrayed as the hereditary degenerate who is feeble-minded or homosexual.

The cult of the superman lay behind the rise of the Nazi party to power in Germany, and it also lies behind the ideas of hereditarian scientists who worry about the children of the poor increasing in numbers faster than the children of the middle classes. This view of humanity sees man as a biological machine remorselessly programmed by heredity, and, as the Nazis showed, it grossly undervalues man.

I would like to offer the hope that human beings may find another, more socially useful vision—the prospect of a new social engineering that seeks to improve people through improving their environment. This vision will put back in our hands, where it belongs, the responsibility for taking political action to change the environment, which, to a great extent, creates us. It is only through understanding who we are and how we got that way that we can hope ultimately to extend the range of possibilities of who we might become.

POLITICS

CHAPTER 1

The Soft Machine: How Genetics Works

The basic facts of biological inheritance are now known to science. Some geneticists may hesitate to say whether intelligence or a predisposition to mental illness is inherited, but they will have no doubts about the inheritance of color blindness or the cause of mongolism. Mongolism was once thought to be an evolutional "throwback" to an earlier Mongolian ancestry, but it is now known to be caused by the presence of one small extra chromosome in the cells of the body. Every cell in a person's body normally contains forty-six chromosomes—the minute structures that carry hereditary information. But due to an accident during the development of the sperm or the egg before fertilization, mongols have forty-seven.

Each of the forty-six chromosomes in the normal human cell consists of a "thread" of deoxyribonucleic acid (DNA), which carries genetic instructions "written" along the length of the thread. The instructions are written in a code within the chemical structure of the DNA—a code with four different "letters." The genetic instructions are decoded by the chemical processes of the cell and translated into proteins that perform various vital jobs.

Some proteins are building blocks from which parts of the growing cells are assembled. Other proteins are enzymes (biological catalysts) which, for example, might break down sugar to yield energy, or build new molecules that are used to form new cells. The code for each of the many thousands of different proteins that can be produced by the cell is carried on small sections of DNA, which are all joined up together in a chromosome. The small section of DNA that exists at a particular place on a chromosome and makes a particular protein is a gene—the unit of heredity. So each chromosome, or thread of DNA, is made up of many thousands of genes joined together. A human being has been estimated to possess about 100,000 genes in each of his or her body cells. Each of us has what the geneticist calls a unique genotype—a unique combination of genes that ultimately orders the development and activity of our bodies. The same genotype, placed in different environments, will develop in different ways because the body develops, adapts, or learns as a result of experience. The result of the interaction of the genotype with the environment is called by geneticists the phenotype. Identical twins have identical genotypes because they have inherited exactly the same genes, but their phenotypes are different because their environments—within the womb and the home—are never exactly identical. When identical twins are separated early in life and placed in different environments, they develop greater differences than if they stay together.

The biological machine is not a hard machine like a steam engine or even an electronic computer. It is a soft machine that can respond flexibly to the demands of the environment. The discovery of the way in which the living cell can adapt its biochemistry to the demands made upon it is as recent as the discovery of DNA in 1953 by James Watson and Francis Crick, and it is almost as important to biologists. One example of the flexible response of the human body is the production of an enzyme in the liver to burn up alcohol or to destroy poisons. A heavy drinker is likely to have unusually large quantities of this enzyme in his liver and so is able to burn up the extra alcohol he drinks more quickly.

About one in fifteen thousand people is albino, with white skin, white hair, and very light blue or pink eyes. These people have inherited defective genes that are not able to give instructions for the brown skin pigment to be made by body cells. They have inherited one defective gene from their father and another from their mother. Most genes are present in body cells as two similar copies; one comes from the father and the other comes from the mother. If only one is defective, the other will usually work well enough to do the job alone. One in seventy people carries a single gene for albinism and has normal skin color, and only if this carrier chances to marry another will they produce one in four albino children, on average. And on average two out of four children will be carriers. The gene for albinism remains masked in carriers because the normal gene is dominant—that is, the normal gene can produce enough pigment to give a normal skin color when it works alone. The gene for albinism, because it is masked by the action of the normal gene, is called recessive.

The difference between normal coloring and albino is the difference between a pigment-making gene that is wholly active and one that is wholly inactive. However, the difference between other kinds of genes is often much more finely graded. Each gene in the cell and each protein it produces may exist in slightly differing forms, causing slight differences in the action of enzymes in the cell and in the development of the body. Except when something goes disastrously wrong, the body as a whole adapts to produce an end result close to the normal human "blueprint." The soft machine can, as it were, be pommeled and pushed into different shapes as it encounters various genetic and environmental influences, so that an almost infinite number of variations can be produced while maintaining the same general pattern. Even when each cell in the body has an extra chromosome, as in mongols, it is possible for the body to develop according to the correct basic pattern—although the result is imperfect.

In each generation the chromosomes and genes are shuffled up and doled out anew during the formation of the sperm and the egg. It is this shuffling of the genetic cards which ensures that each of us gets a unique collection of genes. Another process—mutation—provides new genes by sudden changes that may occur spontaneously or as a result of the effects of chemicals or X rays in the environment. Spontaneous mutations may, for example, occur as a result of a mistake made during the copying of a gene when the cell divides. Perhaps the most famous example of mutation of human genes occurred in the family of Queen Victoria. At least three of Queen Victoria's nine children were carriers of hemophilia, although there was no previous record of the disease in her family. One can be fairly certain, therefore, that the gene arose anew by mutation in her father or mother. Queen Victoria's eighth child, the sickly Prince Leopold, was a bleeder. This was the first hint that she was the carrier of a hemophilia gene, which was later carried by two daughters into other royal families of Europe. Prince Leopold had two children before he died from a minor fall followed by a major hemorrhage. Queen Victoria's two daughters Alice and Beatrice carried the disease into the Russian, Spanish and Prussian royal families.

Hemophilia is caused by a recessive gene that is carried on the X sex chromosome. The sex chromosomes, X and Y, are responsible for the biological differences between the sexes. Women have two X chromosomes and men have one X and one Y chromosome. The gene for hemophilia is carried on the X chromosome and is usually masked in women by a normal X chromosome. But when a man inherits an X chromosome carrying the hemophilia gene it is not masked by the Y chromosome, which does not carry a hemophilia gene, so that man is a hemophiliac and, without modern medical help, might die from a relatively small cut or internal bleeding. The principles by which single genes such as those for hemophilia or albinism are inherited has been understood for about seventy years—since the rediscovery of Mendel's work—and is not the subject of any serious dispute.

Many other human characteristics, such as height, are determined not by one gene but by many genes acting together and are often more subject to environmental influences. People do not fall into distinct categories of tall, medium, and short; there are a few very short people and a few very tall people; most people are somewhere in between. Intelligence, as measured by IQ tests, varies in a similar way.

If two tall people or two people with high IQs marry each other—as they frequently do, for there is often a tendency for like to marry like—their children will tend to be shorter or less intelligent than they are. And if two small people or two people with low IQs marry each other, they will tend to have children who are taller or who have higher IQs. This is called regression to the mean. The reshuffling of genes in each generation is one cause of regression to the mean, but environments are also reshuffled each generation and also contribute toward the regression to the mean. Observation that a characteristic such as height or intelligence regresses to the mean in this way is not sufficient to prove that the character is inherited through the genes. Regression to the mean could be simply the result of variation in the environment. Sorting out how differences between individual people and between races of man are inherited or influenced by the environment is bedeviled by such difficulties.

The various races of man differ in the genes they possess. Some genes are found only in some races, but most are found with some frequency in all races. Despite these genetic differences, all races that have had the opportunity to interbreed have done so successfully. The descendants of mixed races appear to be physically no less healthy than either of the races from which they came. The Hottentots in South Africa are short, with a loose yellow skin, peppercorn hair, and a large rump containing fat deposits. They look entirely different from Europeans but have interbred successfully with them. The descendants of these mixed matings, known in South Africa as "Rehoboth bastards," are taller and probably fitter than either parental stock. This phenomenon is well known to geneticists and is called hybrid vigor. Hybrid vigor seems to be the result of creating new combinations of genes that did not previously exist in either race. New combinations of genes are often better than old ones because they mask recessive genes causing debilitating diseases such as hemophilia or sickle-cell anemia. All races carry such "bad" genes. Sickle-cell anemia, for example, is common among negroes, while the white race carries the Rhesus-negative gene that causes women who carry it and who marry Rhesus-positive men to have "blue" babies. Fortunately this disease can largely be prevented with modern treatment.

When a white and a negro have children, the offspring—known as mulatto—are intermediate in color but have kinky negro hair. If two mulattos have children, a small proportion of them will be like white persons and a small proportion as black as any negro, but most will be some variation of mulatto.

Although it is widely believed that a white and a black person may sometimes have children darker than the black parent, there is no scientific evidence that this ever actually happens. Cases that have been investigated have been found to be either mistaken or the result of illegitimacy involving a darker father. Occasionally, as a result of chance, two light-skinned people with some negro ancestry who pass as whites may have children who look much more negroid. The child may not be darker than either parent, but because of a chance combination of hair and facial features may look negro while the parents look only slightly tanned. This might rarely happen among white South Africans, who have an appreciable mixture of negro genes, but not among white Americans or Europeans, who as a whole have virtually none.

Skin color of negroes is controlled by about five major genes. If negroes and whites freely intermarried in the United States without showing any preference for their own race, the vast majority of the population would be white in appearance after a few generations. United States negroes have on the average about 30 percent white genes and U.S. whites have very few negro genes. Negroes form about 10 percent of the population of the United States. Taking these simplified figures and assuming five genes for skin color, Professor Curt Stern of the University of California at Berkeley has calculated that, after unrestricted intermarriage for several generations, 99.4 percent of the U.S. population would pass as white. The fraction of a percent who were left with dark skin would not, or would only rarely, have other negro features. There is no known biological barrier to a full integration of different races by marriage and interbreeding. So far as is known, the mixing of the genes would be expected to produce healthier and fitter types of man than would be produced otherwise.

CHAPTER 2

Heredity and Politics:
The Rights and Lefts of Genetics

Political misuse of genetics has caused untold misery in both Nazi Germany and Communist Russia. For their own partisan reasons, governments in these two countries have interfered with geneticists and made use of genetics for ideological purposes. Biology and politics meet in the study of human heredity. But too often the meeting of these different disciplines has only brought discredit to both.

Scientists themselves are not blameless. Unguarded scientific speculation by eugenicists—whose prime aim was to improve the human race by selective breeding—lies behind the misuse of genetics in Germany. And in the USSR, politicians exploited the naïve enthusiasm of second-rate scientists to impose ideological restrictions on the entire scientific community. Opposite theoretical attitudes to genetics developed in the USSR and in Germany. Both were unfounded and, in their different ways, destructive.

Nazi Germany preferred a hereditarian-racist position, and the USSR under Stalin preferred an environmentalist one. A sufficient number of geneticists and other biologists supported Hitler's Jewish policy to give it a superficial scientific rationale. These same people provided the eugenic arguments enabling laws to be passed that prevented ordinary Germans from marrying whom they pleased. These arguments ultimately provided the basis for Hitler's euthanasia program in 1939–41 when 80,000 men, women, and children died, apart from the millions of Jews and others who were eliminated on strictly racial grounds.

In the USSR many geneticists were summarily dismissed from

their jobs, and some subsequently disappeared. Books about genetics were destroyed and removed from libraries. Following the ban on genetics in the USSR, the people suffered the imposition of complicated and unproductive methods of agriculture, leading to food shortages and famine. Soviet biology was harmed for a generation or more. Interference in Russian genetics by party politicians centered on methods that they claimed would improve agricultural production.

T. D. Lysenko, an agronomist from a simple peasant background, led the revolt against scientific genetics. He worked his way into an important position as the director of the Odessa Plant Breeding Institute. Ultimately Lysenko became president of the Lenin All-Union Academy of Agricultural Sciences and forced the official adoption of his theories throughout the USSR. He promised quick breakthroughs in agriculture that would improve production. His supporters presented these ideas in a clever ideological way, which appealed to the Party men. Conventional geneticists were abused as "Trotskyite bandits" and "enemies of the people" who were trying to destroy Soviet agriculture by encouraging peasants to sow "elite seed."

Lysenko appeared to believe in the inheritance of acquired characteristics, but his theories were hopelessly muddled. The idea that acquired characteristics—such as the large biceps of the blacksmith—may be inherited was first suggested in the eighteenth century in France by Chevalier de Lamarck. Lamarck suggested, for example, that the giraffe acquired its long neck as a result of physical stretching that was somehow passed on to its offspring. Darwin introduced the idea of the survival of the fittest, but he also made use of some of Lamarck's ideas in a modified form. It was not until after 1900, when Mendel's experiments in heredity were rediscovered, that the distinction between biological inheritance and cultural inheritance of acquired characters began to be understood. Lamarckism was then abandoned as a biological theory in the West but continued to be favored in the USSR and elsewhere as a theory of social evolution. Lysenko attempted to bring Lamarckism back into biology. He believed that one species of plant could be transmuted into another; he thought that wheat might change into rye, barley into oats, cabbage into swedes, and sunflower into strangleweed.

Lysenko rose to fame with claims that he could increase the yield of wheat by soaking it so that it would germinate earlier and thus have a longer growing season. This method had been tried many years before in Russia and had been forgotten. The method was known in the West and is, for example, referred to in the annual report of the

Ohio State Board of Agriculture in 1857 by J. H. Klippart. The method had been forgotten because it was a great deal of trouble and had no practical advantages. But Lysenko used his influence to have the method adopted on a large scale. In some areas, such as the Ukraine, the peasants were encouraged to grow lower-yielding varieties of grain because these were suitable to Lysenko's methods. As a result they were worse off. Ultimately, after years of wasted effort, Lysenko dropped the method.[1]

In Lysenko's hands science took a step back several centuries into an era of alchemy. All his claims were made without any attempt at the kind of scientific proof that is required today. Lysenko's whole philosophy was opposed to the improvement of plant stocks by breeding, and the USSR, which until then had led the world in plant agronomy, fell hopelessly behind. The state chose to back a simple-minded peasant philosophy and elevated it to the status of a science. Anyone who opposed the official line in biology or agriculture was seen as a wrecker and ran the risk of losing his job and his life.

N. I. Vavilov, a Russian agronomist and one of the foremost plant geneticists in the world at that time, was arrested in 1938, along with many of his staff. Vavilov died in prison in 1943. Stalin himself authorized worse purges of scientists in 1948, after promptings from Lysenko. The effects were catastrophic for Soviet science. Many laboratories were disbanded overnight. Professors were dismissed in large numbers, and academic courses rewritten. All genetic literature was removed from libraries, and stocks of fruit flies used for genetical experiments were destroyed. A ban was placed on research in genetics and certain related fields.

For four years all discussion of the issues of Lysenkoism and genetics was censored by both the popular press and the specialist journals in the USSR. The Party line deliberately fostered a Lysenko personality cult. Busts of Lysenko were sold in shops, monuments were built to him, and the state chorus included a hymn in his honor in its repertory.

The extent of this ban on free scientific debate and the fostering of false doctrine is difficult to appreciate in the West today. Lysenko was backed by all the power of an authoritarian state prepared to take arbitrary action. No pressure group of any kind in the West possesses that kind of power. Questions of education and race were a secondary issue in the Lysenko affair and appear to have been used more as a means of discrediting conventional geneticists than as an issue in themselves. Medical genetics was condemned as racist and virtually ceased to exist in the USSR after 1940 until its revival in 1963. All references to genetics were removed from medical courses.

It was in Germany that the racist issue became most disastrously intertwined with politics. The German preoccupation with race and heredity can be traced back at least as far as Calvin and Luther. In the sixteenth century Calvin stressed the idea of predestination and elevated it to a position of the greatest importance in his theology. He began with the observation that there are two categories of men, the elect and the reprobate. Following St. Augustine, Calvin taught that the elect alone are true members of the Church and that they alone would be saved. Whether an individual belongs to the elect or the reprobate is divinely predetermined, and Calvin saw in this the manifestation of the glory of God.

In practice, however, it was impossible to tell whether a particular person belonged to the elect or the reprobate. Therefore, all who had faith in God and in Christ were allowed membership of the Church, except for notorious evildoers and heretics. For the Calvinist, mankind was forever divided by one eternal decision of the divine will. There is a parallel here between Calvin's reprobate and later victims of theories of bad heredity or hereditary degeneration. These latter-day reprobates are homosexuals, the insane, the slum dwellers who suffer from diseases such as tuberculosis, and others who through "indulgence" suffer from venereal disease or alcoholism.

In the nineteenth century, when predestination became the pivot of the new Calvinist doctrine, Nietzsche developed a secular version of Calvinism. Nietzsche saw the human race as if it were suspended on a tightrope fastened over an abyss between animal and superman. In *Thus Spake Zarathustra* Nietzsche exhorts the world: "Could you create a God?—So be silent about all Gods! But you could surely create the Superman. Perhaps not you yourselves, my brothers! But you could transform yourselves into forefathers and ancestors of the Superman; and let this be your finest creating!" [2]

Nietzsche was the son of a Lutheran pastor, and both his grandfathers were ministers. He rebelled against this theology and created a secular philosophy that had many parallels with German Protestant theology. God becomes superman, and divine grace a will to power. Nietzsche believed that the rabble—whom he often called "the bungled and the botched"—might be changed into a nation of supermen by means of this will to power and mastery over self. Selective breeding would also help to achieve this ideal of converting the reprobate into the elect, bad heredity into good.

Nietzsche's superman delighted in warfare and was contemptuous of the "slave mentality" of the lower classes. The Nazis later claimed Nietzsche as an authority for much of their racial philosophy. In the Second World War, Allied propaganda denounced Nietzsche as the intellectual source of Nazi racism. However, both the Nazis and the Allies misinterpreted Nietzsche. Although he was interested in race improvement, he believed—contrary to both Nazi and Allied propaganda—that this should be achieved by racial mixing. Nietzsche assumed incorrectly, as Lysenko did later, that acquired characteristics could be inherited. This was excusable for Nietzsche, since the scientific facts had not then been established, nor had the distinction between physical heredity and cultural endowment been made clear. The Nazis called the inheritance of acquired characteristics a Bolshevik lie. They could not admit any possibility of truth in the idea, since it invalidated their racism. On this issue and on the Jewish issue Nietzsche was totally out of step with Nazi doctrine, although this was disguised by Nazi propaganda.

Nietzsche's books were given the status of holy writings by the Nazis, but they became most widely known through popular interpretations. The Nazis used selective quotations from his books to support their anti-Semitism and their race hatred, not understanding that Nietzsche had denounced anti-Semitism, race hatred, and nationalism. He makes it clear in his book *Human All Too Human* that he believed "the Jew is just as useful and desirable an ingredient as any other national remnant" for "producing the strongest possible European mixed race." [3] Nietzsche wrote of the master race, but for him it meant an internationally mixed race of philosophers and artists who practiced self-control. Nevertheless, the image of a master race and a slave people used by Nietzsche bolstered the philosophy of nazism and helped lay the foundations for the abuse of human genetics and medicine that was to follow.

Philosophers and historians also seized upon Darwin's ideas of evolution to explain the rise and fall of civilizations. In popular versions of evolutionary theory in the nineteenth century, the white man was seen as the greatest achievement of nature, with the negro somewhere between man and ape. Black people were thought to be living fossils. Social theories based on Darwin's ideas provided a scientific rationale for imperialism in the British colonies and for the ruthless extermination of native peoples such as the American Indian or Australian aborigines. Darwin's views were also used to propagate the belief that the middle and upper classes were innately superior and so would win the competition of life. But when it was realized that middle and upper classes had smaller families than did workers, thinkers began to worry that the excessive breeding of the lower classes would swamp society with "inferior" types. Modern society seemed to them to have dangerously ignored the laws of nature and prevented the supposedly beneficial action of natural selection. These are the worries which now preoccupy the present-day proponents of the eugenic and hereditarian thought.

In Germany around the turn of the last century, Ernst Haeckel, professor of zoology at the University of Jena, was the leading scientific exponent of Darwinism applied to man. He deplored the actions of doctors who treated patients who had tuberculosis, syphilis, and mental disease; he believed that these weak and degenerate members of the human race should be left to die. Haeckel thought these diseases were transmitted by inheritance to a great extent and that keeping alive patients with these diseases only promoted the spread of disease to later generations. He suggested that the present generation of the diseased should be eliminated in order to prevent an increase in chronic mental and physical disease.

The influence of Calvinist thought can be seen in Haeckel's proposal that "undesirables" should be examined by a commission that would decide who would be granted "redemption from evil . . . by a dose of some painless and rapid poison." [4] This choice of phrase shows that Haeckel's argument depended as much on theological as biological considerations. Haeckel was one of the most eminent German biologists of the nineteenth century, but if he were alive today he would be considered a blatant racist. His concept of the superman was the tall, blond Aryan type, which he claimed was the ideal human breeding stock. He made his anti-Semitic views quite plain, using his prestige as a biologist to foster his racist views. He founded the Monist League to propagate his ideas and was financially supported by the industrialist Alfred Krupp. Haeckel's theories influenced both Bismarck and the founders of Nazism, and many of his ideas were put into practice under Hitler.

Calvinist ideas of predestination and Nietzsche's idea of a superman laid an ideological foundation for what the Germans called *Rassenhygiene* (race hygiene)—or eugenics, as it was called in England and America. *Rassenhygiene* was well established as an academic study with certain practical aims, such as the sterilization of the unfit and the unwanted, long before Hitler's rise to power. Hitler was not the first to suggest sterilizing the unfit, but he was the man who made it possible politically.

In 1933 the German human geneticists Ploetz and Rüdin—perhaps better described as race hygiene experts—worked on a committee with Heinrich Himmler to prepare laws to provide for the sterilization of the unfit. Hitler's minister of the interior, Wilhelm Frick, was given the job of administering the new laws. When announcing them, Frick said: "The fate of race-hygiene, of the Third Reich and the German people, will in future be bound indissolubly together." [5] This link was publicly acknowledged by human geneticists and race hygiene experts. For example, Professor Otto von Verschuer of the University of Münster—a leading German geneticist—wrote in 1941 in his book *Leitfaden der Rassenhygiene:*

> Decisive for the history of a people is what the political leader recognizes as essential in the results of science and puts into effect. The history of our science is most intimately connected with German history of the recent past. The leader of the German state is the first statesman who has wrought the results of genetics and race hygiene into a directing principle of public policy.

Professor L. C. Dunn, a distinguished American geneticist and a former president of the American Society of Human Genetics, commented in an address to the Society in 1961:

> Although not all geneticists who remained in Germany thus accepted the eugenical and racial doctrines and practices of the Nazis, there is at least evidence that even the serious scientists among them underrated the dangers of the movement until it was too late. From this the melancholy historical lesson can be drawn that the social and political misuse to which genetics applied to man is peculiarly subject is influenced not only by those who support such misuse, but also by those who fail to point out, as teachers, the distinction between true and false science. [6]

Professor von Verschuer replied in a letter to the *American Journal of Human Genetics* that his position had completely changed and he was now opposed to compulsory sterilization for the sake of race hygiene. He said that all intentions of race betterment by means of sterilization should be rejected: the past had given a horrifying example of misused eugenics. He explained how as a simple scientist he had been misled by politics:

> A passage of my book published in 1941 is cited in [Professor Dunn's] address, and I must admit that whenever such statements of my earlier publications are taken out of context and quoted they do shock me today.

I now realize the errors on which such premature formulations were based, and I recognize the possible sources of misunderstanding which I have caused for the reader as well as for myself. I never was a politician. I endeavored to serve only science and I was not an adherent of "enforced race hygiene." It is today obvious and clear for myself that I "underrated the dangers of the movement," perhaps because I was not politically minded.[7]

Nevertheless, hundreds of thousands of people in Germany were sterilized against their will from 1935 until the end of the Second World War. The exact number does not appear to be known but may have reached a hundred thousand or more a year. The ultimate aim was to sterilize about 4 percent of the population. Grounds for sterilization included low intelligence, as measured in an extremely unreliable "intelligence" test. The test included questions such as "Why do children go to school?" and instructions to compose sentences out of the words "soldier," "war," and "fatherland." Other grounds for sterilization included schizophrenia, manic depressive psychosis, epilepsy, blindness, deafness, severe physical abnormality, severe alcoholism, and any supposedly hereditary physical defect.

It was the legal duty of doctors and others to report candidates for sterilization to the proper authorities. A special state doctor (*Bezirkarzt*) then examined the person and made a report, and sometimes obtained a psychiatric opinion. If the patient was dissatisfied with the decision of the *Bezirkarzt,* he could appeal to a higher court. Some curious anomalies showing the impossibility of any fair legal system of compulsory sterilization quickly arose, and these have been described by the distinguished British psychiatrist Dr. Eliot Slater in an article condemning the Nazi eugenic laws.[8]

Dr. Slater describes the case of the daughter of a doctor who had from childhood suffered from an obscure complaint resembling epilepsy, which had increased in severity until she began having major fits. Her father was informed that she would have to be sterilized. He objected and took her from doctor to doctor in an attempt to get her fits recognized as being caused by some nonhereditary factor. Finally a distinguished neurosurgeon diagnosed a brain tumor and operated to remove a large cyst. She recovered completely. In another case a talented musician in Frankfurt suffered from an attack of mania and depression and was ordered to be sterilized. He appealed, and the appeal was granted on the grounds that he possessed unusual hereditary musical talent. For once, these evil laws gave a beneficial result.

Science cannot remain blameless for Hitler's atrocity. Eugenic

theories helped prepare the way for Hitler's policies. The chief German journal of eugenics, *Archiv für Rassen-und-Gesellschaftsbiologie,*
welcomed the idea of excluding Jews from the new German state in an
editorial in the 1930s. A popular textbook called *Human Heredity,*
written by Dr. Erwin Baur, Dr. Eugen Fischer, and Dr. Fritz Lenz,
provides a discussion of the racial psychology of Jews under the guise
of genetics. Fischer was director of the Kaiser Wilhelm Institute for
Anthropology, Human Genetics, and Eugenics. This institute became
so politically involved with nazism that it was abolished after the war
by the West German state. Dr. Fritz Lenz, Professor of Racial
Hygiene at the University of Munich, in his discussion of "racial psychology" suggests that the character of Jews is hereditarily predisposed to revolution—a theory calculated to devalue any genuine political arguments Jews may have had. He says:

> In revolutionary movements, hysterically predisposed Jews play a great
> part, being able to give themselves up unreservedly to utopian ideas, and
> therefore able with a sense of inward sincerity to make convincing prom-
> ises to the masses. . . . The fact that so many leaders of revolutionary
> movements have been Jews is . . . an outcome of the peculiarities above
> described, peculiarities which by no means lead to destruction. Even
> when the Jew destroys, it is usually with the aim of rebuilding.[9]

Lenz then remarks upon "the fondness of the Jews for Lamarckism, that is to say for the doctrine of inheritance of acquired characters." If this doctrine were true, remarks Lenz, the Jews living in a
Teutonic culture would be transformed into genuine Teutons. And this
is why Jews, says Lenz, are fond of the doctrine. However, Lenz con-
demns Lamarckism as an illusion and says that Jews do not transform
themselves into Teutons by writing books about Goethe. Such an
argument as Lenz's presupposes that there are only two possible explanations of the origin of human character: physical inheritance through
the genes (Mendelian heredity) and the discredited inheritance of acquired characters (Lamarckism). However, this totally ignores learning
and cultural endowment as the origin of character differences between
races. The Nazi race theories were made credible by such unscrupulous and unscientific argumentation.
    The German race hygiene laws also interfered with the human
freedom of the ordinary German. Appointments to the state services,
such as the post office, state bank, and railways, as well as the civil
service, the S.S. and the S.A., were given only to Aryans who suffered no hereditary taint (*erblich belastet*). Marriage loans were made

only to couples approved by the state. Certain types of marriage were expressly forbidden by law, and a doctor had to fill in a form before a couple could apply to be married. This included a family history going back to great-grandparents and all their descendants. The doctor then made a diagnosis of race, sanity, hereditary taint, criminality, and any peculiar gifts. Peculiar gifts might include special ability in mathematics, music, art, or languages and also practical abilities, including that for sports. An official decision was then reached as to whether marriage could be allowed and whether the couple merited the marriage loan.

Those with hereditary disorders were allowed to marry only sterile people, and sterile people were allowed to marry only other sterile people or ones with hereditary disorders. People were considered to have tainted heredity if one parent, two brothers or sisters, or a third of other relatives suffered from severe physical or mental abnormality. Even if two quite different conditions such as schizophrenia and cleft palate appeared in the family, the sufferers were added up toward the number who suffered hereditary taint. There is no scientific basis for lumping defects together in this way, and the method used reveals a direct connection with nineteenth-century ideas of bad heredity. Implied in the operation of the Nazi marriage laws was a belief in some general type of hereditary degeneration.

The abuse of eugenics in Germany from 1933 to 1945 cannot be blamed entirely on the Nazis: the ground had been well prepared for them. The responsibility must be shared by those scientists who advocated sterilization and who failed to distinguish between fact and philosophy in their academic teaching of human genetics, race hygiene, and anthropology. These faults were not limited to German eugenics. In America and in Britain and other European countries, scientific standards in human genetics were lowered by the attempt to prove and impose eugenic theories.

German race hygienists looked to Francis Galton, the distinguished English biologist, as the father of their movement. Indeed, there exists some correspondence between Galton and the editor of the German journal *Archiv für Rassen-und-Gesellschaftsbiologie* that shows they agreed together to regard the words *Rassenhygiene* and *Eugenik* as synonymous. Galton's own definition of eugenics was simple enough and not likely to cause any disagreement among German race hygienists. Galton said the aim of eugenics was to give "the more suitable races or strains of blood a better chance of prevailing speedily over the less suitable." [10]

Although Galton cannot be blamed for failing to foresee the abuse of eugenics by the Nazis, he must share responsibility for contributing to the confusion between science and religious philosophy that fed the Nazi racist movement. Galton saw eugenics as a kind of religion based upon science. He wrote:

> There are three stages to be passed through. Firstly it [eugenics] must be made familiar as an academic question until its exact importance has been understood and accepted as a fact; secondly it must be recognized as a subject whose practical development deserves serious consideration; and thirdly it must be introduced into the national consciousness as a new religion.[11]

Galton did not foresee what terrible consequences could follow from such deliberate confusion of science and religion.

Francis Galton will always be remembered as one of the most distinguished biologists the world has known. Although he is less familiar today than his cousin Charles Darwin, he is just as important to the development of modern biological science. He was a pioneer in the studies of meteorology, fingerprints, and statistics. He also laid the foundations of statistical genetics, which is basic to scientific breeding in agriculture today. Genetically, Galton was totally committed to the view that man's life was predetermined by hereditary and environmental forces. He was a determinist and a hereditarian. He recognized that the environment influenced human character, but to him it was almost always secondary to heredity. To Galton heredity was the primary means of predetermination. An inveterate experimenter, he describes in his book *Memories* an attempt to measure his own freewill. Galton's description of this experiment reveals how he saw himself and his fellowmen primarily as automata. With the more rigid social stratification and the more carefully prescribed etiquette of his day, this view is perhaps not so surprising as it is for us now.

However, the very design of his experiment appears to show the existence of a remarkably free and exceedingly curious will:

> I was so harassed with the old question of determinism, which would leave every human action under the control of Heredity and Environment, that I made a series of observations on the actions of my own mind in relation to Free-Will. I employ the word not merely as meaning "unhindered" but in the *special* sense of an *uncaused* and *creative* action. It was carried on almost continuously for three weeks, and on and off for many subsequent months. The procedure was this. Whenever I caught myself in an act of what seemed to be "Free-Will", in the above sense, I checked myself and tried hard to recollect what had happened before, made rapid

notes and then wrote a full account of the case. To my surprise, I found, after some days work, that the occasions were rare in which there seemed room for the exercise of Free-Will as defined above. I subsequently reckoned that they did not occur oftener than once a day. Motives for all the other events could be traced backwards in succession, by orderly and continuous steps, until they led into a tangle òf familiar paths.

It was curious to watch the increase of power, given by practice, of recalling mental actions which, being usually overlooked, give a false idea that much has been performed through a creative act, or by inspiration, which is usually due to straightforward causation. . . . The general result of the inquiry was to support the views of those who hold that man is little more than a conscious machine, the slave of heredity and environment, the larger part, perhaps all, of whose actions are therefore predictable. As regards such residuum as may be not automatic but creative, and which a Being, however wise and well-informed, could not possibly foresee, I have nothing to say, but found that the more carefully I inquired, whether it was into hereditary similarities of conduct, into the life-histories of twins, or introspectively into the actions of my own mind, the smaller seemed the room left for this possible residuum.[12]

Galton's feeling that freewill is so restricted may have derived in part from his own religious background. C. P. Blacker, Galton's biographer, records that Galton was a sensitive and deeply conscientious child and that his awareness of original sin made him feel wretched. Galton records that he felt emancipated from the "intolerable burden of superstition"—meaning his previous religious beliefs—after reading Darwin's *The Origin of Species*. Galton speaks of the book as if it were a baptism that purged him of his oppressive sense of original sin. However, Galton soon developed the idea that sin had natural rather than supernatural origins.

The theology of original sin was replaced in Galton's scheme by eugenics. Following his conversion from religion, Galton saw man's moral nature as having evolved, and he believed that in the future man could control his own evolution and so grow more perfect. Galton believed that negroes have further to go in the evolutionary process than other races. For example, he says in his book *Hereditary Genius* (1869):

The conscience of a negro is aghast at his own wild, impulsive nature, and is easily stirred by a preacher, but it is scarcely possible to ruffle the self-complacence of a steady-going Chinaman. The sense of original sin would show, according to my theory, not that man was fallen from a high estate, but that he was rising in moral culture with more rapidity than the nature of his race could follow.[13]

To Galton the negro was a moral fossil—a missing link in man's moral evolution.

Galton was also opposed to the mixing of the races. He argued that the intelligence of Englishmen was on average two grades—perhaps 20 IQ points as measured today—above that of negroes, and that the intelligence of the "Athenian race" of the fifth century B.C. was two grades above that of a nineteenth-century Englishman. Galton's arguments, supported by numerical evidence, had a brilliant scientific gloss, but his assumptions were dubious or faulty and his actual evidence thin. Galton was simply dignifying with the status of science the popular prejudices held by both biologists and laymen of his day. Galton believed that mixing of the black and white races would decrease the number of people with the highest grades of intelligence. He was opposed to it because, as he says in *Hereditary Genius:* "We know how intimately the course of events is dependent upon the thoughts of a few illustrious men." [14]

Galton classified people according to their "civic worth." There were a small class of "desirables," a large class of "passables," and a small class of "undesirables." He was in favor of diverting material help from undesirables, who he believed monopolized it all, to desirables. Galton also wanted to see the cultivation of an elite class. In 1873 he wrote in *Frazer's Magazine:* "My object is to build up, by the mere process of extensive inquiry and publication of results, a sentiment of caste among those who are naturally gifted." [15] Galton proposed that a biographical index be prepared of gifted families—it was to be a "golden book of thriving families" or "of natural nobility." A volume called *Noteworthy Families* was written and published in 1906. This volume was planned to be the first of a series. Other volumes containing the ancestry of able families were planned, and also a register of families who were notably below average in health, mind, and physique.

Galton hoped that the data for his "golden book" and his blacklist would be provided by a network of local eugenic associations reporting back to a central society. Local professional people would be co-opted to committees that would rate everyone's civic worth. In this way Galton hoped that the "existence of good stocks would be discovered." He hoped that these people of "civic worth" would assist each other in obtaining public appointments. He foresaw a sort of feudal meritocracy where patronage in the form of employment and privileges was dispensed strictly according to inherited "civic worth."

Galton dreamed of a eugenic *corps d'élite*—a caste of superior be-

ings. Galton's superman was the intellectual genius and his Utopia a
Cambridge (England) college. He ended his days elaborating this fantasy in the form of a novel called *Kantsaywhere*.[16] The small state of
Kantsaywhere had a population of only two hundred until a wealthy
benefactor left all his property to a council that was given the task of
improving the human stock of the place. A eugenic college was then
established in the state and a political structure something like an Oxford or Cambridge college set up. Privileges in this society were carefully regulated according to the examination marks obtained by citizens. Those who obtained honors were given special advantages.
Undesirable individuals were to be subjected to surveillance and the
insane or mentally defective segregated from the others for life.

Galton realized that eugenic ideas might be abused if taken over by
an ignorant and unscrupulous dictator. But he cannot have taken this
objection seriously or he would have been deterred from formulating
ideas that were later to be exploited by the Nazis in Germany. Galton's belief in hereditary merit, his enthusiasm for using political
means to improve the "human stock," together with his aim of making eugenics as much a religion as a science, provided a perfect basis
for political abuse.

Despite the work of Galton, opposition to the worst ideas of
eugenics appears to have been strongly based in England. Professor
L. S. Penrose, perhaps Britain's most distinguished human geneticist,
has made clear his view of eugenics in his presidential address to the
third International Congress of Human Genetics in 1966.

> There is one tradition . . . which, personally, I have steadfastly refused
> to follow or endorse. I refer to the cult of eugenics which Galton es-
> poused in the later years of his life. My reason for taking this stand is that
> eugenics is based upon arbitrary valuations of individuals and social
> groups, supported by unjustified and premature assumptions about the na-
> ture of hereditary influences.[17]

Eugenic arguments were used politically with undoubted effect in
the United States between the world wars. Eugenicists, who more
often than not were white and Protestant, argued successfully in favor
of restricting the immigration of "inferior" southern Europeans into
the United States. Harry H. Laughlin, one of the staff of the Eugenics
Record Office at Cold Spring Harbor, was commissioned by the U.S.
government to produce a report on immigration.[18] Using data from the
1910 census when the results of the 1920 census were available,
Laughlin argued that immigration of southern Europeans presented a

threat of social degeneration because such people were innately incapable of being assimilated into American society. As a result of this
report, the U.S. immigration laws of 1924 were based on the national
origin plan, which limited the entry of southern Europeans, among
others, into the United States.

Eugenic arguments were also used to provide reasons for the introduction of sterilization laws, and by 1920 twenty states in America had
adopted them. But the laws were confused in purpose. They often
prescribed sterilization for rapists and sex offenders as well as for the
feeble-minded. Either sterilization was being used as a punishment for
certain types of crime or these types of crime were thought to be hereditary. Other states had laws forbidding the marriage of certain types
of people: the insane, syphilitic, alcoholic, epileptic, criminal, and
feeble-minded as well as people of different race. Many of these
arguments may have been distinctly influenced by the ideas of the
Eugenics Record Office, which had been established in the United
States by Charles B. Davenport, director of the Station for Experimental Evolution at Cold Spring Harbor, Long Island. Davenport believed that members of other races were, in effect, members of different species. He also believed that certain life-styles such as
"nomadism" and "criminality" were inherited as single genes, according to Mendel's laws of heredity. He took a totally hereditarian
view of behavior and was against race mixing because "a hybridized
people are a badly put together people and are a dissatisfied, restless,
ineffective people." [19] Davenport believed that race mixing resulted
in physical incongruities. He used hens as his example. Leghorn hens
have been bred to lay eggs without brooding, whereas Brahma hens
have been bred to lay eggs and then brood on them until they hatch.
The leghorns are suited to chicken farmers who have incubators and
Brahmas to chicken farmers who do not. According to Davenport,
crosses between the two breeds produced offspring that were failures
both as egg-layers and as brooders.

Davenport believed that a tall race of people crossbred with a small
race might produce offspring with "large frames and inadequate vis-
cera." He also theorized that disharmony occurred in mental characteristics as a result of race mixing. He said: "One often sees in mulattos an ambition and push combined with intellectual inadequacy
which makes the unhappy hybrid dissatisfied with his lot and a nui-
sance to others." [20] Other geneticists endorsed Davenport's opinion
and went further in condemning entire races. American eugenicists

Paul Popenoe and Roswell H. Johnson gave biological respectability to racial antipathy in their popular textbook *Applied Eugenics* by saying that racial antipathy had a biological function, that of preventing the races from mixing. They recommended laws not only to make marriage between the races illegal but also to prohibit all sexual intercourse between the races.[21] If these eugenicists had had their own way, the social and political structure of the United States would be more similar to that of South Africa today. In fact fifteen states had laws prohibiting mixed marriages of blacks and whites until 1967, when the U.S. Supreme Court declared miscegenation laws unconstitutional.

The views of geneticists up until the early 1930s were almost universally against the mixing of the races, although there was virtually no scientific evidence to support the view that mixing was bad. It was widely believed, for example, that women of mixed race suffered from a disharmony between the size of the baby's head and the size of the pelvis. The only real evidence produced to support the racial disharmony theory came from Davenport. He studied people of mixed race in Jamaica and concluded that some mulattos had the "long legs of the negro and the short arms of the white, which would put them at a disadvantage in picking up things off the ground." [22] It came out, however, that the disharmony Davenport was referring to amounted to as little as one centimeter in arm length, and in any case Davenport had not investigated a sufficient number of people to be able to be statistically certain of the conclusion.

Other scientists have been unable to find any evidence for disharmony in the physique of people of mixed race. Disproportion between the size of a baby's head and the mother's pelvis is usually the result of malnutrition of the mother in youth. It is still relatively common in countries where the diet given to growing children is poor, but there is no good evidence that it is the result of race mixing.

A study of the descendants of the *Bounty* mutiny who are of mixed Tahitian and English stock shows that there are no signs of racial degeneration among them. This study, made in 1924 by Harry L. Shapiro, who was then attached to Yale University, shows that "the crossing of two fairly divergent groups leads to a physical vigor and exuberance which equals if not surpasses either parent stock. My study of the Norfolk Islanders [where many of the descendants of the mutineers moved from Pitcairn Island] shows that this superiority is not an ephemeral quality which disappears after the F_1 or F_2 generations [the first and second generations of mixed race], but continues even after five generations. Furthermore the close inbreeding which the Norfolk Islanders have practiced has not led to physical deterioration. Their social structure . . . on Pitcairn was not only superior to the society instituted by the Englishmen themselves, but also contained elements of successful originality and adaptability." [23] Other studies of mixed races, which show that mixing of races does not innately have bad physical effects, have been made in Hawaii by L. C. Dunn and A. M. Tozzer [24] and in the United States by Melville Herskovits. [25]

Darlington writes: "The worst results [of crosses between different races] arise in man in such situations as Tristan da Cunha and Pitcairn where the genuine F_2 situation arises." [26] (The F_2 situation arises when members of the second generation intermarry, as they must do on a small island, rather than marrying back into one of the ancestral races.) Darlington neglects, however, Shapiro's evidence and now appears to stand virtually alone among established scientists in his opinion.

In the 1930s Dr. Fritz Lenz was still able to say categorically in *Human Heredity* that "the crossing of the Teuton and Jew is likely, as a rule, to have an unfavorable effect, for it will impair the peculiar excellences of both types." [27] But as Hitler rose to power and began to act on the theories that academics had previously endorsed, a reconsideration of genetic theories of race began—at least in Britain and the United States. There was no real change in the evidence available for scientists to use in formulating theories, but there was a noticeable swing in scientific opinion, first toward neutrality and later even toward favoring race crossing as possibly beneficial. Scientists recognized the threat to personal liberty inherent in Nazi doctrine. For the first time they foresaw the consequences of their theories and began to change them. Scientists did not at first come out and say that the races were equally well endowed by nature, but for the first time they encouraged a questioning of beliefs and a search for new evidence. Distinguished biologists such as Julian Huxley and J. B. S. Haldane began to say that the evidence necessary to decide the question of race crossing just did not exist.

In 1951 UNESCO issued a statement endorsed by some fifty eminent anthropologists and geneticists showing that science could provide no evidence that might lend any support to race prejudice. It stated: "As there is no reliable evidence that disadvantageous effects are produced thereby, no biological justification exists for prohibiting intermarriage between persons of different race." [28] And: "Available scientific knowledge provides no basis for believing that the groups of mankind differ in their innate capacity for intellectual and emotional development.'' [29] The publishing of these statements marked an almost complete reversal of accepted scientific opinion. The reversal had taken place slowly over a period of some ten or fifteen years. However, comments made by geneticists at the time and published by UNESCO showed that many were not prepared to agree with the second statement. Professor William B. Provine, a historian of science at Cornell University, Ithaca, New York, commented:

> Few geneticists wanted to argue, as had the Nazis, that biology showed race crossing was harmful. Instead, having witnessed the terrible toll, geneticists naturally wanted to argue that biology showed race crossing was at worst harmless. No racist nation could misuse that conclusion. And geneticists did revise their biology to fit their feelings of revulsion. [30]

Professor Provine believes that geneticists' ideas about hereditary differences in intelligence between races may now be undergoing another change, so that the majority of geneticists will eventually agree with the second UNESCO statement. He says:

> In 1951, judging from the response to the UNESCO second statement on race and comments in genetics literature, most geneticists agreed . . . that races probably differed in significant average mental traits. By 1969, when Arthur Jensen advocated this view in his controversial article, most geneticists who spoke publicly on the issue had adopted an agnostic position. Knowledge of hereditary racial differences in IQ had scarcely changed since 1951, but society had changed considerably in racial attitudes. [31]

The intellectual problems and many research programs in eugenics arose before genetics became a science. Thus early work in eugenics was based on ideas that proved to have no general validity. This weak intellectual foundation, which included the bad-heredity concept, has carried over into human genetics, and has influenced the course of research long after the ideas themselves have been largely abandoned.

However, the idea that social decay is caused by bad heredity of one kind or another seems to be too strong ever to be entirely dispelled. As recently as 1973 Konrad Lorenz, who was awarded the Nobel Prize for his studies of animal behavior, revived the idea that society is suffering from genetic decay. Lorenz believes that hereditary behavior patterns are responsible for an innate sense of justice in some people and an innate tendency in others to commit crimes. Lorenz sees ''progressive infantilism and increasing juvenile delinquency'' as signs of genetic decay that is spreading like a ''malignant growth.'' He says:

"There is no doubt that through the decay of genetically anchored social behavior we are threatened by the apocalypse in a particularly horrible form." [32]

When people look for certain guidance in the face of explosive social issues, science is sometimes used to give authority to what people want to believe anyway. Experts are consulted, and when hard evidence is scarce, the experts who can produce answers in the spirit of the times are most readily believed. This process of appraisal may occur outside the regular stream of evaluation of scientific ideas, yet it can carry as much influence as genuine science. History shows that genetics has been used repeatedly in this way, and in subsequent chapters we will see that it is still being misused in the current debates about intelligence, sex, crime, and health.

CHAPTER 3

Are We Slaves of Inheritance?

A man may easily produce 200 million sperm in one ejaculation. Each of these sperm is unique, and each of the 300 or so eggs that a woman's body produces during her reproductive life of twenty to thirty years is also unique. Egg and sperm unite to give the fertilized egg a unique combination of genes. The result is that each person is an individual unlike any other. Is the character and fate of each of us decided at this moment of conception? Attempts to answer this question have caused one of the most bitter disputes ever to divide biologists.

One school of thought, the hereditarians, believe that intelligence is 80 percent inherited. They would argue that other qualities, such as musical ability, mathematical ability, and personality, are strongly inherited too. They would say, in effect, that people's lives are decided at the moment of their conception, and so each person's struggle to live the way he or she would like is primarily a struggle with his or her own hereditary limitations.

The argument continues with the assertion that the majority of poor people are poor because they are not intelligent, and that the majority of the children of the poor will also be poor, whatever advantages they may be given, because intelligence is 80 percent inherited. Heredity provides a convenient explanation for such differences between people, which otherwise might only be accounted for as the result of social privilege. This is because any difference that is inherited tends to be regarded as an individual's own good or bad fortune; no one else is to blame.

Hereditarians justify privilege on the grounds that the majority of the privileged are of a superior hereditary type. Blacks, women, the poor and sick, they say, are physically or mentally inferior and that is why they tend to occupy a lower social position. At the extreme, hereditarians would divide us all up into social castes prejudged as to ability and performance.

One such present-day caste theory of society has been proposed by Richard Herrnstein, professor of psychology at Harvard University. He says in his book *IQ in the Meritocracy* that, as social class barriers fall and the environment becomes more uniform, heredity will become increasingly important. He believes that ultimately people will be born as "alphas" and "gammas" just as anticipated by Aldous Huxley in *Brave New World*. He says:

> As the wealth and complexity of human society grow, there may settle out of the mass of humanity a stratum that is unable to master the common occupations, cannot compete for success and achievement, and is most likely to be born to parents who have similarly failed.[1]

Herrnstein concludes that a more egalitarian society cannot be achieved by "greater wealth, health, freedom, fairness and educational opportunity." He believes that those who strive for an egalitarian society will achieve the opposite—a society sharply graduated into castes.

Herrnstein's thesis is only the latest in a long series of hereditarian theories that have been used to attack egalitarian principles. Hereditarians have attempted to explain history in terms of biology. C. D. Darlington, professor of botany at Oxford University, England, has based a major book, *The Evolution of Man and Society*, on this theme.[2] Darlington states his thesis in an earlier book, *The Facts of Life:* "The materials of heredity contained in the chromosomes are the solid stuff which ultimately determines the course of history."[3] Darlington also believes that each person has a preordained position in life. He goes on: "Individuals and populations cannot be shifted from one place to another after an appropriate period of training to fit the convenience of some master planners, any more than hill farmers can be turned into deep sea fishermen or habitual criminals can be turned into good citizens."[4]

Darlington's speculations are based on a popular view of man. This is the evolutionary view that in societies simpler than our own the most intelligent men and women are able to support the largest number of children and so contribute most to the next generation. A constant obsession of this school of thought is that people with inferior IQs are pampered and encouraged to have large families by social welfare and so are lowering the intelligence of future generations.

This view of our society is based on dubious biology and ultimately on social and scientific prejudice. Heredity is without doubt of great importance in deciding the form and function of our bodies and all its organs. But the brain is an exceptional organ, different in kind from all other organs of the body. Its function is dependent upon learning—it is not simply a machine programmed by heredity.

Opposing the hereditarian ideal is the environmentalist school of thought. Environmentalists argue that many important human characteristics, including intelligence, personality, and health, are profoundly influenced by the environment. The disagreement between the two schools is profound because of the implications for society. Human beings cannot at present alter their heredity; they can alter their environment. If the hereditarians are right, then all efforts to improve the environment by investing in education and health will yield diminishing returns. But if the environmentalists are right, then shrewd investment in improving social conditions and in education will increasingly improve the standard of life for all.

The early environmentalists were as incautious in pushing their views as the hereditarians. John B. Watson, the leader of behaviorist psychology, boasted in 1924, "Give me a dozen healthy infants, well-formed, and my own special world to bring them up in, and I'll guarantee to take any one at random and train him to become any type of specialist I might select—doctor, lawyer, artist, merchant-chief, and yes, beggar and thief, regardless of his talents, penchants, tendencies, abilities, vocations and race of his ancestors." [5] No one today would claim to be able to do this, although the time may not be far off when we will understand how children come to develop specific abilities and finally choose a vocation. Until recently little was known about the ways in which the development of children could be influenced under the age of five. But now new methods of teaching children under five, which involve the parents as aides in the school, are showing promising results. Deprived children from poor slum families are able to develop above-average intelligence as a result of some of these programs.

J. McVicker Hunt, professor of psychology at the University of Illinois, makes a modest and realistic assessment of an environmentalist's hopes today:

At this stage of history, it is extremely important that both political leaders and voters understand the limited nature of our knowledge about how to foster competence in the young, that they understand the basis for our justified hopes, and that they comprehend the need for the continued support of fundamental research and of the process of developing an adequate technology of early childhood education. Only with continued support for research and development in this domain can we expect to create effective means of compensating for and/or preventing the deficiencies of early experience required to meet the twin challenges of racial discrimination and poverty.[6]

The biological facts of human heredity do not lead irrevocably to the hereditarian thesis. Taken together with the psychological researches of men such as Mc Vicker Hunt, they justify another, more noble view of man. As the United States Declaration of Independence states: "We hold these Truths to be self-evident, that all Men are created equal." This has often been taken simply to mean that all men should be given equal opportunities. But the fathers of American independence are right in a deeper sense. Children from deprived backgrounds whose parents have depressed IQs can do as well as or even better than average—that is, they can achieve IQs above 100—if they are put in a favorable environment at an early age. Biologically we are all unique individuals, but given the same chances we would all be much more equal than most people think. But is a genuine increase in equality politically possible? The battle rages as science and ideology become means to political ends.

When Arthur Jensen, professor of educational psychology at the University of California at Berkeley, published his views on genetics and education in the *Harvard Educational Review* in February, 1969, he was accused by students and academics of racism and elitism. The furor reached such a pitch of anger, and Jensen at times felt in such danger, that he was forced to leave home to hide in a hotel under an assumed name. Jensen's offense was to disturb cherished notions about the basic equality of man. He had—or so he believed—spelled out the scientific reasons why backward American negro children were doomed to failure because of their inherited deficiencies in intelligence and educational ability.

Similar accusations and harsh treatment have been given to Professor Hans Eysenck, professor of psychology at the Institute of Psychiatry in London, and Professor Richard Herrnstein at Harvard. Their lectures have been disturbed and canceled at the last moment. In 1971 Eysenck wrote a book supporting Jensen, and shortly afterward he was punched and spat at, and had his spectacles broken by angry students. Students have threatened to stab Professor Herrnstein after a lecture, and campus police have said that they were unable to guarantee his safety.

Jensen's academic arguments provoked taunts and insults. Pamphlets were distributed at Berkeley bearing a photograph of Jensen with the title: "Hitler is alive and well and spreading racist propaganda at Berkeley!" Students went so far as to ask the university's Board of Regents to fire Jensen. At Harvard, students circulated a poster with Herrnstein's photograph and the words: "Wanted for racism. Richard Herrnstein (alias Pigeonman)." The poster detailed the charges as "the fraudulent use of science in the service of racial superiority, male supremacy and unemployment."

Such personal attacks and physical threats are unusual in academic life. They are dangerous signs, which show a failure of professors and students to communicate at all levels. At first sight the fault appears to lie entirely with the students who have failed to listen. But the professors are not innocent. They command their audiences as eminent experts on a subject where expertise is most vulnerable to prejudice. And the more certain our experts are that their discipline is above prejudice, the more vulnerable they are to it.

Jensen, Eysenck, and Herrnstein share a basic presumption that heredity plays a primary role in shaping society. Although there are important differences between their views, the central point of agreement is that IQ is 80 percent inherited and of overwhelming importance for success in life. They view attempts to compensate for deficiencies of intelligence by special teaching and welfare programs as a waste of time and money. They see egalitarian ideals as impractical in the face of the realities of heredity. In effect, they appear to believe that human nature is largely predetermined by heredity, the environment relatively unimportant, and freewill severely limited. This is the hereditarian position—the odds for or against people are spelled out in their genes and, except for accidents, they are predetermined to become officers or men, slaves or supermen, as their genes prescribe. Between them, these three professors have seemed to condemn the American negro, the Australian aborigine, and the native Irishman as innately inferior in intelligence.

"Genetic slavery" is one of the recurring themes of hereditarians. For example, Arthur Jensen asks in his article in the *Harvard Educational Review:*

Is there a danger that current welfare policies, unaided by eugenic fore-sight, could lead to the genetic enslavement of a substantial segment of our population? The possible consequences of our failure seriously to study these questions may well be viewed by future generations as our so-ciety's greatest injustice to negro Americans.[7]

Jensen believes that children in the lower socioeconomic groups of society often lack the genetic heritage that would enable them to learn through understanding, and he advocates the greater use of rote learn-ing in instructing these children.

Richard Herrnstein states these same fears. In his book *IQ in the Meritocracy*, Herrnstein develops his theory that people are being sorted out into hereditary castes. Before long, Herrnstein says, "if and when technology has truly replaced the drawers and hewers and the other simple vocations, the tendency to be unemployed may run in the genes of a family about as certainly as the IQ does now." [8]

Professor Herrnstein believes that, as society becomes more com-plex, inherited IQ will become more important for success. At the same time he predicts that there will be an increasing tendency for like to marry like, with the effect that society will separate out into biologi-cal castes. These castes, unlike those of the past or present, will be based on genetic superiority and so revolution will not be easy. Herrn-stein sees this sort of heredity meritocracy as inevitable and says, "We should be preparing ourselves for it instead of railing against its dawn-ing signs." [9]

Similar fears have been voiced by William Shockley, Nobel laureate and professor of engineering at Stanford University, who has warned of the deteriorating "human quality" of the population of the United States. Shockley asks similar questions to Jensen:

The FBI records show that between 1962 and 1967 violent crimes per capita have risen at more than 10 per cent per year. The intensity of riot violence has been increasing even faster; my best estimate of the trend for the last five years is a compound interest growth rate of about 50 per cent per year. The central question that I pose in respect to these trends is this: Do these indications of deterioration of the quality of our national social behavior have as an underlying cause the possible decline in the quality of the U.S. population? [10]

Shockley also fears a future of "genetic slavery." He says: "The available facts lead me to fear that illegitimate, slum birth rates are lowering negro hereditary potential for intelligence so that the result may be a form of genetic enslavement that may provoke extremes of racism with resultant misery for all our citizens." [11]

The hereditarian school of thought is concerned not only with color but also with social class. Hans Eysenck makes this clear in his book *Race, Intelligence and Education,* which is written as an ardent defense of Arthur Jensen. Eysenck says that "one important reason for the existence (and composition) of the 'lumpenproletariat' . . . may be the genetically determined low intelligence of those who have descended into it." [12] Eysenck also considers that "mental illness, criminality and personality generally have strong roots in genetic constitution" [13] and gives these as other reasons for the existence of the lumpenproletariat. He adds that bad luck and "in some cases" color prejudice may also contribute to a person's descent into the lumpenproletariat. Eysenck is basically committed to the idea that the lower classes, the criminals, and the mentally ill occupy their place in society because of hereditary disadvantages. The hereditary disadvantages listed by Eysenck—low intelligence, mental illness, and criminality—are among familiar components of the nineteenth-century bad-heredity concept.

The concept of bad heredity was well established in a semiscientific form before the science of genetics began with the rediscovery of Mendel's laws of heredity in 1900. The bad-heredity theory suggested that a whole complex of debilitating conditions, which it is now easy to see are associated with poor living conditions, are inherited. Tuberculosis and syphilis were then considered to be hereditary in the same way as hemophilia is known to be inherited today. Included in this idea of bad heredity were "the criminal instinct," insanity, feeble-mindedness, and immorality, which included prostitution and homosexuality. Incredible though it may seem today, even pauperism was considered to be a sign of bad heredity: there is nothing new in the idea that the poorest classes are destined to be genetic slaves. It was even said that such characteristics as left-handedness, stuttering, use of foul language, and being hunchbacked were the result of bad heredity.

The idea that language is directly influenced by heredity is still maintained by C. D. Darlington, who says, "Race builds language. And language builds race." [14] And other scientists today have an unshakable belief that predisposition to criminality, homosexuality, alcoholism, drug addiction, and mental illness—particularly schizophrenia—are inherited, though the scientific evidence is full of uncertainties.

There are social if not political advantages to be gained by the established classes in encouraging the belief that human intelligence, health, and character are prescribed by heredity rather than acquired during life. If, for example, the predisposition to tuberculosis were inherited, then society could more easily have ignored the conditions of overcrowding in slums that caused the prevalence of the disease in Europe up to twenty or thirty years ago. Since improvements in housing and modern drugs have enormously reduced the incidence of tuberculosis, it is no longer politically important whether or not a predisposition to the disease is inherited, so it is easier now to assess the scientific evidence objectively.

Similar issues are still hotly debated with reference to, for example, schizophrenia. If schizophrenia could be shown to be inherited, then we could all be excused from making an agonizing reappraisal of the strains of family life, which may yet be found to be the most important cause of the condition. Belief that mental illness is inherited has also served to justify the policy of segregating the sufferers in large asylums where they will not breed and will not bother the rest of us.

Belief that criminality is inherited can be used to justify long prison sentences for the recidivist. If the full logical implications of the inheritance of a criminal predisposition were accepted, it would remove the fundamental notion of our law that a person is responsible for his or her actions unless found to be insane.

The use of tests to detect children who might later become criminals was seriously considered by President Nixon in 1969. Dr. Arnold Hutschnecker, a New York psychiatrist who treated Mr. Nixon for what was described as a "physical complaint" in the 1950s, proposed to the President that six-year-olds in the United States be tested to determine their potential for future criminal behavior. Dr. Hutschnecker recommended that the criminal tendencies of six-year-olds be tested using the Rorschach method, which judges a person's reaction to a set of standard ink blots. And he suggested that massive psychological and psychiatric treatment be given to those children found by this means to have criminal inclinations. The scheme was sent by President Nixon to the U.S. Department of Health, Education, and Welfare for evaluation and was shelved after a negative report. Dr. Hutschnecker's idea of finding the cause of crime within the minds of individuals, rather than in the evil circumstances of the world we live in, gains strength from the idea that a predisposition to crime is strongly inherited.

The belief that homosexuality is inherited is popular for slightly different reasons. If homosexuality is thought of as an inherited condition similar to the color of a person's skin, then homosexuals are seen as a race apart and their behavior, otherwise incomprehensible to the heterosexual, is neatly explained. If this explanation is accepted, it is then easier for extreme factions to deny homosexuals the same consideration as the rest of society. And homosexuals themselves are often ready to believe in a hereditary theory of homosexuality because it provides an easy explanation of their feelings—and once they believe that their "fate" has been decided, it must be easier to adjust to it.

A related issue is whether women possess an inherited femininity or motherliness that makes them happy to play a subservient role in society. Is this subservient role women's natural fate? Are women genetic slaves? The assumption frequently made by men in the past that women are genetically predisposed to enjoy subservient roles is now being challenged by women, so that men are again beginning to marshal scientific evidence to prove their superiority.

The woman's liberation movement compares the status and role of women in society to that of racial minority groups and by analogy has identified the prejudice against women as sexist. Science is perhaps even more subject to such sexist bias than to a racist bias. Kate Millett, one of the first women in the modern struggle for women's rights, says in her book *Sexual Politics:*

> Each of the social disciplines contributed to re-establishing and then maintaining a reactionary status quo in sexual politics, each through its own method of reasoning: anthropologists might study cross-cultural divisions of labor and ascribe them to a fundamental biological source, while sociologists, in announcing that they merely recorded social phenomena, gradually came to ratify them by noting that nonconformist behavior is in fact deviant and produces "problems." The psychologist, in deploring individual maladjustment to social and sexual role, finally came to justify both as inherent psychological nature, fundamental to the species and biological in essence. Later this point of view acquired sufficient confidence to go on the offensive.[15]

Science has been used to rationalize a sexist view of marriage, the family, and women's role in society.

Biological science has often been used to attack the classic notion that human beings are rational and free. John Stuart Mill, the great English advocate of liberty, wrote: "Of all vulgar modes of escaping from the consideration of the effect of social and moral influences on the human mind, the most vulgar is that of attributing the diversities of conduct and character to inherent natural differences."[16] White domination of a large part of the world is based on this simple premise, and the class

52   *Who Do You Think You Are?*

structure of society is similarly based. White supremacy is ultimately
justified by theories that whites are innately superior at abstract thinking and that the average black has childlike thinking processes. When
the theories of Jensen, Eysenck, and Shockley are placed in this context, the difficulties of achieving scientific objectivity in discussing inheritance of IQ can be seen more realistically. The difficulties go far
beyond those usually encountered in scientific inquiry.

Biological theories of heredity have also been used to support the
idea of aristocracy based on exclusive marriages and good breeding,
when what is really being inherited is property or social position.
Theories of hereditary excellence have been used to justify the idea of
an intellectual meritocracy of scholars and scientists.

Present-day studies of the inheritance of intelligence have been directly inspired by the work of Francis Galton and his lifelong study of
genius. In 1908 Professor J. Arthur Thomson, a distinguished zoolo-
gist and not an immoderate man, said that Galton's studies of hereditary genius gave us "a biological pride of race and a respect of true
aristocracy." [17] The same sentiment lies behind much of the argument
about the inheritance of intelligence today, although it is not expressed
in such forthright terms.

It is justifiable to ask if there is any real scientific value in all the
observations made about the relationship between heredity and IQ.
The effort has been great, but the scientific reward is still small because major difficulties of interpretation remain. Is it of any *scientific*
importance to know whether the negro inherits genes that give him an
inferior IQ or to know the exact degree to which a white man's intelligence is inherited? Some scientists believe that the theoretical scientific interest of these observations is negligible. Then why have Jensen, Eysenck, Herrnstein, and Shockley undertaken such arduous
work?

To consider motive and sentiment may appear to some unscientific
in itself. Jensen, Shockley, Herrnstein, and Eysenck have all complained that the arguments about heredity and environment have often
become lost in personal accusations and what is called the *argumen-
tum ad hominem*—an argument appealing to personal prejudice rather
than reason. However, it is legitimate to ask why scientists and a particular school of science choose to ask certain questions and not others. Science is influenced by the mood of the age and the preconcep-
tions of scientists. The questions that scientists interested in heredity
have neglected to ask are as important as the ones they have chosen to
ask. For example, until recently, identical twins were studied pri-

marily in attempts to measure how heredity influenced a characteristic and seldom as a means of identifying factors in the environment that may have influenced that characteristic. The reason for this was simply that identical twins were studied primarily by scientists with a genetic leaning who were not interested in analyzing environmental factors.

There has been another important trend that has influenced scientific thinking about intelligence, mental illness, and crime. Genetics is a science that is capable of great precision and has an elaborate and engaging theoretical basis. It has proved irresistible to those psychiatrists and psychologists who look for a model of the human organism defined in terms of physics and chemistry. Genetics appears to be the first logical step in this reduction of man to physics and chemistry. Once heredity is invoked, otherwise incomprehensible observations appear to become predictable. In recent years this philosophical commitment to reductionism, rather than any simple political motivation, has been a predominant scientific driving force behind hereditary theories in psychology and psychiatry. This trend of thought, joining with the tangle of nineteenth-century ideas about bad heredity and racial inferiority, has provided the basis for much hereditarian psychology.

The fatal scientific weakness in the hereditarian view of humanity is its lack of evidence. The history of the subject shows that the method of using human twins to measure hereditary influences contains hidden assumptions. One of the most basic difficulties, for example, has been to obtain samples of twins that are unbiased by social class. As the dangers of bias from studying twins selected in an arbitrary way became appreciated, greater efforts were made to obtain something approaching a random sample. However, because of the great difficulty of obtaining twins separated shortly after birth, this is virtually impossible to do. A study of twins published by Sir Cyril Burt in England in 1966 [18] is considered by Jensen to be one of the most valuable of all studies of inheritance of IQ because the twins came from a wide range of social classes. But, this study contained another important potential source of systematic error. Only one of each twin pair was actually adopted, usually by relatives, and the other remained with its natural parents. It is useless to argue that the environments of these twins are independent—even though Burt showed that the occupations of the fathers were not correlated—when the foster parents are known to be related to the natural parents. All too many studies of the heredity/environment problem are made possible only by allowing such assumptions, which beg the very questions at issue. A scientific resolution of the debate will be possible only if these difficulties of method are fully faced and if they can be solved—which is by no means certain.

In the meantime, hereditary theories of human nature continue to lend theoretical support to the idea of an inevitably stratified society of slaves and supermen, geniuses and toilers, whites and blacks, officers and enlisted men. No one seriously denies that genetical differences must exist between types and classes of men. The question at issue is whether the extent of these differences is generally of any importance compared with people's ability to learn and to adapt to new ways.

It might be possible for science to provide the objective evidence that would settle the controversy between those who believe that human nature is predetermined by heredity and those who believe in the importance of the environment and freewill. In theory, science might indeed settle the issue with relevant evidence. However, science has not yet expurgated itself sufficiently from ideology to be able to give a clear answer.

SEX

Perhaps the most important lesson we all have to learn in life is how to function in our sexual and social roles as men and women. We may fail at school, or we may be relatively unsuccessful in our careers, and still find happiness in family life. But if we fail to learn how to function effectively in our sex lives and in our male or female roles in society, then misery and torment often follow. Our conditioning to think male or think female is usually so strong that it does not always occur to us to question the influence of it on our lives. If we are to begin to understand who we are and what made us the way we are, we must first question how we function in our sexual relationships and in our family life. In the chapters that follow, I try to sort out what part, if any, of our sex roles is fixed by heredity and what part is learned through our experience of human relationships, so that we can begin to distinguish those differences between the sexes which are truly innate, those which are our own private obsessions, and those which are forced upon us by society. This is the first step toward a new freedom to be what we want to be.

CHAPTER 4

Sex and Intersex: The Biological Facts

Neither male chauvinists nor radical feminists will find much to comfort them in the biological facts about sex. A few years ago it was still possible for both sides to find arguments from biology and psychology that appeared to support their case. Within the last five years, science has come nearer than ever before to understanding the elusive factors that create not just the physical but also the psychological differences between the sexes. And the answers are unexpected.

Babies in the womb are literally brainwashed by hormones that prepare them for the sexual roles they play in later life.[1] Although a person's genetic sex is decided at the moment of conception, the fetus begins to develop in the womb in a basic sexless pattern from which the male or female anatomy develops under the influence of hormones. Those same hormones cause irreversible changes in the brain of the fetus that influence a person's sexual behavior throughout his or her life. But how many of us are truly 100 percent male or female? Most people take their sexuality for granted and have no doubts about whether they are male or female. However, whether the sexual criteria invoked are anatomical or psychological, there is a spectrum of types ranging from totally male to totally female.

Only a fraction of 1 percent of babies are born whose sex is so doubtful that medical tests are necessary to establish whether they are male or female, but it is these unfortunate individuals who provide clues that show how the rest of us are all varying mixtures of the two sexes. Another 10 percent of people who are homosexual live on the psychological borderline between the sexes.

For most of us, the need to question which sex we belong to never

arises. But the following bizarre examples of confused sexuality will
show how complicated the distinction can become in certain rare
cases.

Sport is one area where women will probably never compete
equally with men. Men are stronger and larger and are more often
prepared to train with total dedication. Sportswomen—like women
doctors and scientists—give scores in psychological tests of feminini-
ty/masculinity that are much closer to men's than to those of other
women. Indeed, some sportswomen are more "male" according to
such tests than are some male artists and musicians. Women with
masculine physiques are likely to do best in most women's sports.
Until new international rules and sex tests prevented it, some of the
best world-class competitors in women's athletics events were intersexes. "Intersexes" are people who exist in the no-man's-land between man and woman: their bodies are partly male and partly female.

On September 15, 1967, Ewa Klobukowska, the Polish athlete,
was ruled ineligible for the Women's European Athletics Cup competition in Kiev after failing to pass a sex test. She was shattered. Previously she had been co-holder of the world record for the 100-meter
sprint and winner of gold and silver medals at the Tokyo Olympics in
1964. A board of three Soviet and three Hungarian doctors found that
she had "one chromosome too many" and ruled that she was not to be
allowed to compete as a woman in international athletic competitions.
Ewa Klobukowska was the first person to be disqualified under a regu-
lation requiring sex tests for women athletes competing in international
events. These tests involved a full medical examination of the body as
well as a test of the chromosomes. Miss Klobukowska was a case of
borderline sex: she had previously passed conventional medical tests in
Budapest in 1966. Six months after the Kiev ruling, the International
Amateur Athletic Federation decided to withdraw ratification of all
Miss Klobukowska'a medals, and her name was struck off the record
books of athletics. She probably suffered from Klinefelter's syndrome—a chromosome condition causing abnormal sex development—but this has never been publicly admitted.

The true sex of many other women athletes will never be known
for certain. Until the European Athletics Championships held in Budapest in 1966, athletes needed only a medical certificate signed by a
doctor in their own country as evidence of their true sex. A full visual
examination was introduced in 1966, and the chromosome test in
1967.

The simple visual examination was sufficient to discourage four champion Russian athletes from appearing at the meeting. Gabriel Khorobkhov, leader of the Russian athletics delegation, admitted, "We have left behind some athletes because, like any other country, we have borderline cases. We want to save them any possible embarrassment." [2] Most famous of the Russian athletes of doubtful sex were Tamara and Irina Press. Tamara held the world record for the shot put and Irina was the Olympic pentathlon champion. The true circumstances of the sex of these girls is not known, but they were certainly some kind of intersex.

Borderline cases have been causing trouble in women's athletics since the 1930s, although it is only recently that the problem has been at all well understood by doctors. In 1938, when Hitler was pushing for records at the European Championships in Vienna, Dora Ratjen broke the women's high-jump record with a leap of five feet, seven inches. Later she had an operation and changed her name to Hermann. Hermann took a job in a restaurant and was nicknamed the "Hamburg waiter" by the world press. His world record was struck off and the British girl Dorothy Tyler was awarded the title.

At least one woman athlete, Claire Bressolies, French 100-meter sprinter who competed for her country in 1952, has fathered children following a sex-change operation. She must have possessed all the essential male organs before the operation, but the appearance of the organs must have been superficially female because of a quirk of development.

Behind these curious facts lies human tragedy. A person who is unsure of his or her sex will always be insecure. Some intersexes cannot be assigned with certainty to one sex or the other. In the past, doctors and midwives, as well as laymen, did not understand the problems. Sometimes the sex of a baby was decided with a quick glance at birth and no one questioned the decision until doubts were raised at adolescence. Intersexes—men and women whose true sex is a matter of doubt—are also called hermaphrodites. The word comes from the Greek myth about the son of Hermes and the goddess Aphrodite who became fused in one body with the nymph Salmacis. Some hermaphrodites have male chromosomes and glands, together with the outside appearance of a female, while others appear to be males equipped with a penis and scrotum, but inside, all their organs are female, and at puberty their breasts begin to grow. Only about one in five hundred people is of doubtful physical sex, but these rare individuals show how the male and female forms are the extremes of a basic pattern laid down in the developing fetus.

Doctors recognize at least four different ways of deciding a person's sex. First of all, there is the obvious method of looking at the appearance of a person's external genitals. Second, tests can be made on body cells to find out what chromosomes a person has. Third, it is important to know what internal sex organs—ovaries or testes—a person has, and this requires exploratory surgery of the body. The final factor in judging a person's sex, and the most difficult to decide, is the psychological one. A person's psychological sex may be quite different from his or her physical sex. Some people are so unhappy as a member of their own sex that they are prepared to mutilate their genitals or commit suicide rather than continue to live as they are. They are utterly miserable with the sex into which they were born and sometimes will go to great lengths to obtain an operation to change their sex.

The sex of body cells is decided at the moment of conception when the sperm fertilizes the egg. It is a beautiful but deceptively simple process. Normally, women have two X chromosomes in each cell of the body, whereas men have one X chromosome and one Y chromosome. But, as in the case of Miss Klobukowska, mistakes sometimes happen and the body may be formed with more or less than the usual number of sex chromosomes. When body cells have the wrong number of sex chromosomes, then sex organs will often, but not always, develop in an intermediate way. But even when the number of sex chromosomes in each body cell is correct, the sex of the growing embryo may develop incorrectly if hormones coming from the mother enter the baby's body via the placenta in abnormal quantity. This may happen when one of the mother's hormone-producing glands is overactive.

The growing embryo does not show any sexual features until the buds of the sex glands (ovaries and testes) appear. In the human embryo this occurs at the age of seven weeks. The external sexual organs begin to develop later from basic structures that are common to both male and female embryos. Each structure in one sex has an equivalent at some time during development in the other sex. The clitoris of the female is, for example, equivalent to the penis in the male, and males have nonfunctioning nipples and a small structure called the uterus masculinus, which is equivalent to the womb.

People who suffer from the rare condition called Turner's syndrome have only one X chromosome and no Y chromosome. These individuals often have no internal sex organs, but they have the external genitals of the female. They are underdeveloped sterile females, a condition resulting from the fusion of a sperm lacking an X or Y chromosome with a normal egg or from the fusion of an egg lacking an X chromosome with the sperm carrying an X chromosome. (A normal man is XY, a normal woman XX, and an individual suffering from Turner's syndrome is XO, where O means no chromosome.) In the absence of a Y chromosome there are no clear genetic instructions to develop as a male, and so the body develops in the female direction. To develop as a normal female the human embryo must have at least two X chromosomes and no Y chromosomes in the majority of the body cells. An extra Y chromosome will cause the embryo to develop in the male direction. Individuals with two X chromosomes and one Y chromosome—the condition known as Klinefelter's syndrome—develop as males, although they are sterile and have a small penis and testicles. They also have some female characteristics: scant body hair and some breast development. A larger than expected proportion of them are mentally subnormal, but some have normal or high intelligence. They always have a low-powered sex drive, which cannot be increased by injections of sex hormones. The existence of such people with too many or too few chromosomes shows that it is normally the Y chromosome that is responsible for causing male sex organs to develop in men and produce male hormones.

However, people with Y chromosomes do not always develop as males—some develop as attractive women with well-developed breasts who are to all appearances normal. Their internal sex organs—the womb and sometimes the vagina—fail to develop normally and testes are concealed within their bodies. Genetically these women are males—every cell in their bodies is male—but they develop as females. This condition is called the testicular feminization syndrome.

Until women with testicular feminization consult a doctor because of sterility, sexual problems, or failure to have normal monthly periods, they do not know that they are in any way out of the ordinary. Sometimes women who have this syndrome have a very small vagina or perhaps no vagina at all, but seldom discover this before their first sexual relationship. However, a vagina may be created surgically in a number of different ways. One way is to use a small piece of intestine. Recently a woman in Greece who suffered from this condition had a vaginal transplant. The organ was donated by her mother, who was a widow and considered that she had no further use for it. The vagina is relatively easy to remove surgically as a muscular tube some five inches long. The mother who donated her vagina would of course be unable to have sexual intercourse or to have more children, because what had been the entrance to her vagina was sewn up surgically. Although a transplant may at first seem the ideal solution (if someone can be found who can spare this organ), it means indefinite maintenance on drugs to prevent rejection of the transplant.

Women who have the testicular feminization syndrome have probably inherited a gene that causes them to convert the male hormone testosterone into the female hormone estrone. Normal women have small quantities of testosterone circulating in their bodies, but women with testicular feminization have none. This perhaps accounts for their ultrafeminine appearance and attractiveness, which is so often remarked upon and is probably due to especially well developed breasts, a clear skin, and extremely little body hair.

When doctors discover by means of chromosome tests that a woman has the testicular feminization syndrome, they usually do not tell her exactly what it is. It would make no sense to tell a woman who has no doubts about her femininity that her cells are totally masculine and that she is the victim of a mistake in heredity. It would only make her feel insecure in a feminine role to which she has become emotionally adjusted. If asked a direct question, a doctor ought to answer truthfully, but he should try to avoid telling patients distressing and irrelevant facts about their condition.

Sympathy with the position of women who suffer from this syndrome led a group of Danish doctors and scientists from Aarhus University to object to the sex tests for women athletes in the 1972 Olympics. They pointed out that appalling psychological damage could be done to a woman if it was suddenly revealed that she was genetically male. However, their objection was not successful, because if sex tests had been abandoned the way would have been open for women with an extra Y chromosome and a more masculine physique to compete unfairly. What seems to be needed is a more flexible set of rules for international sport that would allow women with the testicular feminization syndrome to compete as normal women, since they have no unfair physical advantage. The objection to this is that intermediate stages of testicular feminization exist where women do have a more masculine, athletic body build. As always, the problem is where to draw the line. The present rules seem to provide the best compromise until better tests are devised.

Normal men who consult their doctors because they may have a hernia or because only one of their testes has descended are sometimes found to contain female organs in their bodies. On operation the surgeon finds a uterus, fallopian tubes, and inactive ovaries. These cases can be explained only by a failure of the testes in the fetus to produce the hormone that inhibits growth of the female structures. Despite their ambiguous anatomical sex, these men are able to marry and appear to have a normal sex life, although they may be sterile.

Development of the male baby may go wrong when there is a deficiency of the male hormone testosterone at the critical stage when the external genitals are developing. One result of this is hypospadias, an intersexual condition where the opening of the bladder to the outside is not placed normally at the end of the penis but may be in the female position or anywhere on the shaft of the penis. This often means that a boy with hypospadias—unless it is a mild case—can urinate only in a sitting position until a surgical repair is made. Often associated with hypospadias is the failure of the skin of the scrotum to fuse in the middle, which leaves the testes in two separate pouches, sometimes with a short vaginal pouch in between. When these abnormalities are extreme they cannot be distinguished from the testicular feminization syndrome.

These cases of hypospadias have often been assigned to the wrong sex in the past. Provided the penis is large enough to begin with, it is always possible to make repairs by plastic surgery, and the condition is completely curable. If the penis is only a little larger than a normal clitoris, however, the child is unlikely to become a well-adjusted male, whatever his genetic and developmental sex really is. In the past it has not been possible to predict reliably whether a child with hypospadias will develop breasts or not at puberty, or whether he will be able to function as a fertile male when the male sex organs are fully restored by surgery. If unwanted breasts do develop at puberty, these can always be removed surgically.

It is now possible to test whether the phallus of an intersexual infant will respond to hormones as a clitoris or as a penis. Dr. John Money, medical psychologist and eminent sex researcher at the Johns Hopkins School of Medicine in Baltimore, has found that if the infant phallus responds with sexual excitement to the application of male hormone cream, the infant will probably respond sexually as a male.[3] Those that do not respond in this way are probably cases of incomplete testicular feminization and will be better raised as females even though they have typical male chromosomes. A penis can always be modified by plastic surgery into a clitoris, and further hormone treatment may be necessary in adolescence. However, before these tests were available it was frequently found that people with hypospadias were able to adjust well to whatever sex, male or female, they were assigned at birth.

One cause of hermaphroditism in genetically female babies is an unusual activity of the adrenal gland (the so-called adrenogenital syndrome). Instead of producing the hormone cortisone, the adrenal gland of the baby within the womb produces a hormone that has a masculinizing effect. The effect does not occur until after the ovaries and internal reproductive organs have been formed, so it is only the external organs and perhaps the brain that are affected. In extreme cases, there may be a normal-looking penis and a small scrotum containing no testes, but more often there is simply an enlarged clitoris and a normal vagina. If left untreated, children with the adrenogenital syndrome may develop premature male sexual characteristics with the growth of pubic hair in infancy. This syndrome can have a variety of causes but can often be treated by hormones or surgery to give the person the appearance of a completely normal, fertile woman.

When the penis is fully formed at birth, these children can be raised as males, and they can learn to identify fully with the male sex. However, when the condition is recognized early, they are readily converted by surgery into girls, although Dr. Money observes that they have less than the usual interest in doll play and have tomboyish traits.

The sooner surgery is carried out, the better, so as to prevent any ambiguity of upbringing. Doctors believe that when surgery is delayed and the parents are doubtful about the sex of their child in the early years, the child is more likely to have doubts about its sex role in later life and perhaps ask for a change of sex. This shows that a person may develop psychologically as either sex if there is doubt about his or her anatomical sex. But when parents are uncertain of the sex of their child they may treat the child ambivalently and so cause the development of profound doubts in the child's mind about his or her sexual identity.

It is relatively rare for hormones to have an abnormal effect in the womb on the physical development of sex. Effects on the developing brain of the fetus could be more common and could have the effect of blurring the hard edge of the psychological division between the sexes. Very rarely is the sexual development of the brain totally at odds with the rest of the body. When that does happen, a woman's brain with its natural sexual preferences is trapped within the body of a man, or a perfectly formed woman may have a man's sexual preferences. In such extreme cases it may be easier to change the body by surgery than to attempt to change the mind. People who seek these operations have ususally lived for some years as members of the opposite sex and do not respond to psychotherapy. They are desperate to change their bodies and sometimes mutilate themselves in pathetic attempts to change the body they hate. The tragedy of these people and the medical, social, and legal difficulties they face in changing their sex are just beginning to be appreciated now that some thousands of people throughout the world have had their sex changed surgically.

CHAPTER 5

Brainwashed by Sex and by Gender

The bizarre story of April Ashley, who, before a sex change operation, was merchant seaman George Jamieson, has made legal history. In 1963 in Gibraltar April Ashley married as a woman and in 1970 was sued for divorce. The judge, Mr. Justice Ormrod, who is also a doctor, granted the divorce with a ruling that April Ashley was not a woman, although he agreed that she was a male transsexual, possibly with some minor physical abnormality. Mr. Justice Ormrod said, "She is not a woman for the purposes of marriage, but is a biological male and has been so since birth." [1]

April Ashley was born a man with normal male chromosomes. At the age of twenty-four he started to take estrogen hormones and his breasts began to develop. He then had a sex-change operation in Casablanca, and an artificial vagina was constructed. He had led a miserable life as a man and several times attempted to commit suicide. Doctors at the Walton Hospital, Liverpool, described him as a "constitutional homosexual," but he always maintained that his only aim was to live as a woman. After the operation, she was so successful as a woman that she was able to establish a career for herself as a fashion model and was in great demand. She modeled women's clothes in many magazines, including *Vogue*. But then *The People* newspaper revealed that she had originally been a man, and she was no longer able to get work.

In 1963, at the age of twenty-seven, April Ashley married Arthur Corbett, son and heir of Lord Rowallan, a former British Chief Scout. Their marriage took place in Gibraltar, but lasted only a few days and was never consummated. When Mr. Corbett sued for divorce in 1970 it was the first case in which an English court had been asked to consider what is meant by a person's sex and to define sex for legal purposes.

Mr. Justice Ormrod maintained that Miss Ashley's sex-change operation could not affect her true sex: "The only cases where the term 'change of sex' is appropriate are those in which a mistake as to sex is made at birth and subsequently revealed by further medical investigation." [2] The judge said that for the purposes of marriage the criteria of sex must be biological. He argued that even the most extreme degree of transsexualism in a male or the most severe hormone imbalance that could exist in a person with male chromosomes, male sex organs, and male genitals could not create a person who was "naturally" capable of performing the essential role of a woman in marriage.

The failure of the marriage did not occur simply because it had not been physically possible to consummate it. Doctors who examined Miss Ashley found that there was no impediment to sexual intercourse, and Miss Ashley said later that she had had successful intercourse with others. However, Mr. Justice Ormrod held that Miss Ashley was physically incapable of consummating a marriage because sexual intercourse using the "artificial cavity" created by surgery could not possibly meet the legal definition of "ordinary and complete intercourse." He said that such intercourse was the reverse of ordinary, and in no sense natural. "When such a cavity had been constructed in a male, the difference between sexual intercourse using it and anal or intra-crural [between the legs] intercourse was, in his Lordship's judgment, to be measured in centimetres," [3] the *London Times* Law Report solemnly recorded on February 3, 1970.

The judgment left April Ashley in a legal limbo. She had legally changed her name by deed poll and had been issued a woman's national insurance (social security) card, which enabled her to work as a woman. She had also had her passport changed, but she was unable to persuade the Registrar-General to change her birth certificate. Legally she is, and probably always will be, a man.

The Lancet, the medical weekly, commented on the legal dilemma of transsexuals highlighted by the April Ashley case. It said in an editorial that an authoritative tribunal with legal recognition was needed to decide on the question of a person's sex. The tribunal should have a lawyer as chairman, and other members should include a psychiatrist, an endocrinologist, and a gynecologist. It went on:

Requests for reassignment of sex could be made to this tribunal, whose final decision, after carefully sifting all the evidence, would be legally binding. An essential requirement would be the acceptance that registration by the tribunal carried with it all the rights of the re-registered sex including employment, pay, pension rights, inheritance and marriage. So long as the Law stipulated that there are only males and females it is irrational to register an individual as one or the other and then attempt to place limits (so far as that person is concerned) on the rights accorded to that particular sex.[4]

If a tribunal of experts, such as that proposed by *The Lancet*, is ever formed, it would have to decide how important people's psychological sex is relative to their anatomical and genetical sex. Mr. Justice Ormrod avoided this issue by considering only what is legally female *for the purposes of marriage*. By this device he conveniently bypassed the vital question of how a person's sexual identity is determined. This may be a question of little, if any, legal significance, but it is absolutely fundamental to understanding the causes of the differences between ordinary men and women.

Before a transsexual person, such as April Ashley, has had a sex-change operation, his or her anatomical sex is unambiguous. Biologically such people are born as perfect anatomical specimens. Why, then, do they want to change sex? Are there subtle differences between the way they are reared and the way normal children are reared? Or are there subtle differences in their biological makeup that have hitherto defied detection by science? Does the suggestion that a person has a psychological sexuality separate from his physical sex have any validity?

Transsexuals have an overpowering desire to live full lives as members of the opposite sex. They dress in the clothes of the opposite sex and may be able to establish lives for themselves as members of the opposite sex—in some cases after an otherwise successful marriage with children. Dr. Martin Roth, president of the Royal College of Psychiatrists, records one extraordinary case of a transsexual who came with a request for surgery:

> One of our patients was a petty officer of 49 years who wore women's underwear including a roll-on corset and silk stockings throughout the Second World War as the chief petty officer of a cruiser. At the height of the war in the Mediterranean he rented a room on shore where he could in solitude dress entirely in women's clothing when on leave. The ambition to achieve a change of sex by surgery was said to have been lifelong.[5]

Transsexualism is sometimes thought of as the extreme of transvestism. Transvestites, however, have no wish actually to live as members of the opposite sex and often dress up in clothing of the opposite sex simply to obtain erotic excitement. Transsexuals are also quite different from homosexuals. Homosexuals are not normally interested in dressing up in the clothing of the opposite sex and would be as disturbed at the idea of a change of sex as anyone else. Unlike homosexuals, transsexuals usually have a low libido, and if they have any sexual experience prior to their sex change it is seldom homosexual.

Children reared as boys will usually prefer to remain boys, and girls prefer to remain girls, even when their sexual anatomy is in disagreement with their social sex role. Dr. John Money quotes several cases to illustrate this conclusion: one girl with a large and visible phallus was well adjusted to a feminine role; two boys with exceptionally small penises and poor male features nevertheless had strong feelings of masculine identity. In these cases environmental conditioning seems to be more powerful than heredity in deciding the child's sexual identity. Many women who have a very masculine appearance due to the adrenogenital syndrome, which causes the clitoris to develop into a penis and hair to grow on the chin, have no wish to become male despite their male appearance, and despite the fact that they have far greater amounts of male hormone circulating in their bodies than normal men do.[6]

Occasionally a hermaphrodite with hidden testes who is reared as a girl asks for a change of sex in later life. In these cases it looks as if a basic masculinity is forcing its way out, perhaps because the brain is sexually male. Doctors are naturally sympathetic to these cases because they cannot deny that the person was born biologically male. However, most hermaphrodites of this kind are happy as women. They would probably be unhappy as men because they only have small, inadequate penises, which cannot as yet be improved upon by medical or surgical treatment.

Thus the evidence suggests that intersexes who, biologically, are neither fully male nor fully female are very much influenced by the way they are brought up. It has been argued from the example of such intersexes that normal men and women also adopt the sexual roles they do because they have learned them during childhood. But the weakness of this argument is that it uses the pathological case to explain the norm. If a person is an intersex, it is understandable that the environment might tip the balance one way or the other, but these same influences may have quite different consequences for a normal person. Study of transsexuals and of experiments with animals suggests that hormone influences on the brain before birth are also of great importance. Biologists call this phenomenon the "sexualization of the brain." It can be thought of as an irreversible brainwashing by sex hormones.

Psychiatrists now distinguish between sex and gender. The heterosexual man and the homosexual man both have biologically male sex and masculine gender, but the transsexual man has male sex with feminine gender. At its simplest, sex is what people appear to be biologically, whereas gender is what they feel they are regardless of anatomy or chromosomes. Sex is the result of the anatomical processes of development determined by genes on the chromosomes. Gender is now being explained as the result of hormone effects on the brain in infancy or before birth, and of learning a sex role from parents and others. "Gender is like language," says Dr. Money. "Genetics ordains only that language can develop, not whether it will be Arabic or English." [7]

Most transsexuals have long and miserable struggles to establish a place for themselves in life and often come to the notice of doctors after attempted suicide or threats of suicide. They are obsessed with the idea of living as the opposite sex. In the case of male transsexuals, they occasionally manage to castrate themselves or mutilate their genitals in attempts to remove the male organs they find so offensive. About three or four times the number of male transsexuals come to the notice of doctors as of female transsexuals. This is perhaps because it is easier for a woman who wants to dress in masculine clothes and lead a male type of life to do so. A man who wants to look feminine and be a housewife is regarded as mad, whereas it is only perhaps odd for a woman to dress in male clothes, and it is easier for a woman to find a job where male dress is acceptable.

Some transsexuals are content just to live as members of the opposite sex, even when their appearance as members of that sex is peculiar and unconvincing to others. However, most male transsexuals say they feel much happier after taking estrogen tablets, which usually cause some development of the breasts. Estrogen therapy also has the effect of reducing male libido, which may in itself be beneficial for transsexuals, because it reduces their feelings of sexual conflict.

The removal of the male genitals would be an inconceivable desire for a normal man. It violates a deeply held taboo and is associated in most men's minds with their deepest fears. Most women feel similarly about their breasts. But these organs which are objects of some pride for the normal person are objects of hate for the transsexual, who feels trapped inside a body of the wrong sex. Transsexuals are often extremely persistent in their desire for surgical removal of their sexual organs and are said to resist all attempts at psychotherapy. Unlike hermaphrodites, who are born incomplete as either male or female, transsexuals are physically more or less normal, and so surgeons rightly hesitate to operate.

A request for a change of sex from male to female tends to be most sympathetically considered by doctors, simply because it is technically much easier to change a man by surgery into a woman. No one has yet successfully created a fully functional penis by plastic surgery. There have been some passable imitations. One artificial penis created by a London surgeon was stiffened with a piece of rib bone, but it did not prove successful in action. Many transsexuals of female biological sex are enormously relieved simply to have their breasts removed. This enables them to live and work as men with much less chance of being discovered, which is all that some transsexuals want.

Dr. Harry Benjamin has closely followed the results of surgery on ninety-five male transsexuals and thirty female. He says the results have been good in one third of the patients, satisfactory in another third, and definitely unsatisfactory in less than 10 percent.[8] Occasionally mistakes are made. Transvestites or homosexuals who persistently take the female part occasionally pass themselves off as transsexuals—perhaps thinking it will please their partner. They have the operation and later regret it. Doctors usually insist that a transsexual live successfully for at least two years in the adopted sex before surgery is agreed to—otherwise tragic errors can be made. There have now been a thousand or more sex-change operations performed in the world, at least six hundred in the United States alone.

Several theories have been proposed to account for transsexualism. Most remarkable of all, because of its failure to account for the facts, is Freudian theory, which was formulated in the days before sex-change operations had been performed. Freudian theory does not distinguish between transvestites and transsexuals. Freudians have made the incredible suggestion that transvestism is a method of overcoming castration anxiety! Freudians believe a man, by dressing as a woman, is able to cope with his fear that his father wishes to remove his sexuality, which at the extreme means castration. The extraordinary aspect of this theory is that it assumes that male transsexuals most fear what we now know they most desire and will go to great lengths to obtain— that is, castration. Transsexuals seem to be the only group of men who do not fear castration.

Transsexualism might be caused by childhood envy of the opposite sex, but the facts do not easily fit this suggestion. However, most boys express a preference for their own sex. Transsexualism might be expected to be commoner among girls than among boys if purely social and psychological processes were most important. But in fact it is much commoner among men than among women. This might be explained by boys having special problems in learning their sex roles. Boys are predominantly reared by women during their formative years and may sometimes have too little opportunity to study the male role. At some stage, boys must switch from modeling themselves on their mothers to modeling themselves on their fathers. The difficulty of making this switch when the mother is dominant and the father unhelpful is one possible social and psychological cause of transsexualism and homosexuality.

There is some evidence that transsexuals do have parents who provide inadequate models for children to imitate. Professor Martin Roth [9] found that a dominant mother was even more common among the parents of transsexual men than among the parents of homosexual men. He also found that transsexual men more often had poor relationships with their fathers than did homosexuals or neurotic men. But Dr. Roth was able to find no really convincing differences between the childhood experiences of transsexuals and homosexuals that would suggest that the difference between their favored sex roles arose either biologically or as a result of subtle childhood influences.

Dr. Virginia Prince, an American sociologist, is a transvestite of male biological sex and edits a magazine for transvestites in Los Angeles. Smartly dressed in sweater and skirt, she told a London conference on gender identity in 1969 that male transsexualism, transvestism, and homosexuality may arise from boys identifying with different aspects of womanliness. [10] According to this view, a homosexual emulates the sex role of the mother or some other female figure, whereas the transsexual man emulates the psychological and emotional role of a woman. The transsexual primarily seeks feminine gender rather than female sexuality. He is interested in thinking and feeling as a woman. Finally, Dr. Prince suggests that the transvestite emulates the social role of a woman. A common cause of all these various sexual identities could be different types of unsatisfactory relationships with parents combined with abnormal influences of hormones on the development of the brain in the womb.

The sexual behavior of all animals is controlled by the pituitary gland at the base of the brain, which is in turn controlled by the hypothalamus, a part of the brain itself. The pituitary gland sits snugly next to the hypothalamus and receives directions immediately from it via a special blood supply. It controls the sexual cycle in animals and menstruation in women. When male hormones coming from the testes sexualize the brain of the young male animal, they abolish this cyclical pattern of hormone secretion in the pituitary. Female hormones allow the cyclical pattern to develop.

A young female rat treated with a single injection of a male hormone shortly after birth remains anatomically a perfect female with vagina and uterus but never develops the normal female cycle and does not come into heat as a normal female would. Such masculinized females behave like males: they will mount other animals and make thrusting movements with the pelvis as if attempting intercourse.

Although normal female rats occasionally make thrusting movements, masculinized female rats do it habitually. The female sexual role cannot be restored to these animals by giving them injections of female hormones later in life. A single injection of male hormone in early life has an irreversible effect on the brain.

If male rats are castrated at birth, and so not exposed to male hormones during the critical period shortly after birth, they develop a female behavior pattern, with a hormone cycle and willingness to accept a mounting male at the appropriate part of the cycle. Yet these male rats have a completely normal male anatomy and could not be distinguished from normal males except by analyzing their hormones or observing their behavior. These effects are also irreversible. This is what Professor Alfred Jost of the University of Paris calls the "sexualization" of the brain. The profound effects of a single injection of hormone came as a great surprise to scientists, who had previously thought of hormones as acting more slowly over much longer periods of time.

Sexualization of the brain occurs only at a brief period near the beginning of life. If a male rat is castrated later, the effect is quite different. The rat will then behave as an undersexed male, but nevertheless a male. The situation is similar in the female rat. Once the brief period of sexualization of the brain is over, a single injection of male hormone will have little or no permanent effect.

Although it is impossible to prove conclusively, the human brain is almost certainly sexualized by hormones in a similar way. Rarely a person may be born whose sex organs and brain are sexualized in different directions, because of a change of hormones in the body of the mother or in the fetus itself. The change in hormones circulating in the mother and fetus could possibly be caused by stress or the effect of disease on the glands of mother or baby. In humans the brief period when the brain is sensitive to sex hormones occurs while the baby is still in the womb. This is because humans are born at a relatively more mature stage of development than rats. The sensitive period for sexualization of the brain in human pregnancy probably occurs between the 60th day and the 120th day.

These experiments show that it can be misleading simply to deduce a person's sex from chromosome tests and anatomical examinations. It is not true that, once the genetic dice have been cast, the matter is settled and someone who refuses to accept his or her genetic sex—or even his or her anatomical sex—is refusing to accept the facts. Chromosome tests can take no account of the unexpected effects of the environment on the development of the embryo or the peculiarities of psychological development up to puberty.

There are few opportunities actually to test whether anything similar to sexualization of the brain occurs in humans, but such evidence as there is suggests that it does. Women who are threatened with early miscarriage may be given synthetic progestin (pregnancy hormone) to help save the pregnancy. Occasionally this hormone may have a masculinizing effect on a female baby, so that the external genitals are slightly or even strongly male. This condition is easily recognized, and corrective surgery can be performed in early infancy, so these girls need never know that their sex was once ambiguous. Dr. John Money reports examining nine of these girls to discover if the hormone exposure had had any lasting effect on their behavior. He found no evidence of repudiation of their sex role or of lesbianism in these nine girls, but he did find that most of them were interested in outdoor athletic activities with vigorous energy expenditure and were often known as tomboys. They tended to prefer boys' toys to dolls and also to prefer a casual unisex type of clothing. They also gave priority to their careers over having families, or at least expected to combine the two. Taken together, these observations suggest that the hormone exposure may have caused them to develop a more masculine life-style, although they were still well within the normal feminine range.

Experiments with animals show how the effects of stress on pregnant mothers may upset their normal hormone balance and interfere with the normal sexualization of the brain of the baby. There is no reason to believe that the human hormone-producing glands would react to stress in a fundamentally different way. Dr. Ingeborg Ward, a psychologist at Villanova University, Pennsylvania, exposed pregnant rats to stress from a bright light in a confined space. The male offspring of these mothers showed very feeble sexual behavior. Few of them attempted to mate when presented with a receptive female, although, when they did mate, they performed normally. These male rats were then castrated and injected with female hormones. They were then found to be much more ready to allow themselves to be mounted than castrated rats that had not been exposed to stress in the womb. This confirmed that the brains of these male rats had been sexualized in the female direction as a result of the stress on their mothers while they were in the womb.[11]

One of the effects of stress is to cause the adrenal glands to produce more hormones, including two male sex hormones, testosterone and androstenedione. The androstenedione is a much weaker male hormone, but it acts on the same sites in the body as does testosterone. When a pregnant animal is exposed to stress, these two hormones will pass from the mother's circulation into the circulation of the embryo. The result, shown in these experiments, is that male rats whose mothers are exposed to stress while they are in the womb will become less male, while females will become more male.

It seems likely that this effect of a stressful environment on the adrenal glands may be no evolutionary accident but rather a natural way in which the size of animal populations is regulated. Overcrowding causes animals great stress, and as a result their adrenal glands increase in size, influencing the ability of later generations to reproduce themselves. An extraordinary experiment conducted by Dr. John Calhoun at the National Institute for Mental Health in Bethesda, Maryland, shows that this may happen in a population of mice when overcrowding occurs and the young mice cannot move away. The experiment was deliberately designed to have features similar to those in existing cities where it is difficult for the young to escape to a new life. If the fate of the mice provides a valid comparison, and if life becomes more stressful, it seems possible that there will be an increase in the numbers of people who are psychologically caught between the sexes.

Dr. Calhoun started his mouse colony, called Universe 25, with four breeding pairs. There was enough food and water in the colony for at least 6,000 mice, but the population never exceeded 2,200.

When it reached this peak after less than two years, there were still spare nest sites that were not being used. At first many mice lived to an age of over eight hundred days—equivalent to eighty human years. But within four years, despite a constant supply of food and water and the absence of any disease, the colony died out. The mice were unable to live together in what Dr. Calhoun designed to be a mouse Utopia.[12]

Trouble began when after eighteen months the new generation of young males could find no *Lebensraum* and so could not escape from the colony to found new communities. This generation turned to mugging and sexual assault. Tension increased in mouse Utopia and the mothers started to neglect their young. The next generation of mice—which Dr. Calhoun called "the beautiful ones"—were passive and withdrawn and could not perform sexually. Gradually breeding in the colony came to a total stop and the last generation of mice died of old age without having had offspring. When young, these mice had been unable to develop any adequate emotional bonds with their mothers, and they may also have been subjected to unusual hormone experience while in the womb. Whatever the actual cause, hormonal or social, this experiment shows in a frightening way how the environment can influence the young and totally alter normal social and sexual patterns of behavior. Dr. Ward's experiments may provide an explanation of what happened in Universe 25. The mice that Dr. Calhoun called "the beautiful ones" may have been made sterile and passive as a result of exposure to androstenedione in the womb. Dr. Calhoun's experiment shows how under these artificial conditions stress can destroy a community by literally making it impotent. To argue directly from mice to men is always hazardous, but in this case there may be a valid comparison. People also respond to stress by alteration of hormone output in their bodies, and people also require a secure home territory in which to "nest." Women are often more placid and accepting during pregnancy, but when they are harassed at this time they may batter and kill their unborn babies. Other distressed mothers may simply neglect to feed or care for their children. A harassed mother, living perhaps in one room in an inner-city block, is likely to have children who are passive and withdrawn until they grow up, when they may turn to violence. We do not know if these children are likely to have ambivalent sexual behavior resulting from abnormal hormone exposure in the womb. Such stress during pregnancy could be one of the factors influencing some people to become transsexual or homosexual, but there are other social factors that are also—perhaps more—important.

CHAPTER 6

Homosexuality: Destiny or Preference?

Two popular myths—neither of which is true—encourage the belief that homosexual men are not biologically male but are destined by heredity to be different. First, many people believe that homosexuals seldom change their sexual habits in later life, and second, many people believe in the existence of a recognizable homosexual type. However, there is no real evidence to suggest that the effeminate behavior of the homosexual who advertises his homosexuality is in any way instinctive. Rather, it seems to be behavior that is learned and has the purpose of helping the homosexual acquire a mate. The everyday behavior of many homosexuals is quite indistinguishable from that of heterosexuals. A homosexual is simply someone who prefers to have a sexual relationship with a member of the same sex.

The only way homosexuals can be reliably distinguished from other people is by using a lie detector technique. A male homosexual who is shown pictures of men will unconsciously dilate his pupils or show a momentary change in the electrical resistance of his skin, due to a change in blood flow, whereas he will not react in the same way to pictures of women. The latest refinement of this technique is to attach a special rubber band to the penis and use this, coupled with electronic instruments, to measure changes in the size of the penis. This technique, known as phallography, has been used in at least one Eastern European country to diagnose homosexuality in men in order to avoid enlisting homosexuals for army service.

Measurements of the size of homosexuals' bodies, the proportions of their hips to their shoulders, and the distribution of their body fat or body hair have totally failed to find any difference between homosexual and other men. Psychological tests show that homosexual males, like heterosexual males, vary from the feminine to the masculine in their vocabulary and interests. Personality tests have failed to distinguish homosexuals from heterosexuals unless they contain items referring to sexual situations.

About 4 percent of men are exclusively homosexual throughout their lives, according to the results of the famous Kinsey survey of four thousand American men. Surveys on smaller numbers of men in other countries suggest the same figure. Kinsey also found that up to 25 percent of men were occasionally homosexual, and that one man in ten has a period of at least three years during which he is exclusively homosexual. Many more men may have homosexual feelings that are carefully suppressed.[1]

The idea that homosexuality is inherited has persisted ever since Victorian times, when Freud endorsed the idea and was supported by his eminent contemporaries Havelock Ellis and Krafft-Ebing. Perhaps the idea persists because it provides everyone with a convenient explanation and can be used to mitigate the powerful social pressures on homosexuals to change. Homosexuals themselves often prefer to believe that their nature is decided by fate acting through their inheritance. This absolves feelings of guilt and may relieve anxiety that might follow from a search for emotional causes.

Some psychologists take an uncompromising view that homosexuality is a basic inherited factor in the personality. Hans Eysenck said, "The evidence is very strong that homosexuality has a very marked genetic component."[2] And C. D. Darlington has been another keen advocate of the view that homosexuality is hereditarily determined. He also supports the view, which has never been satisfactorily sustained, that homosexuals of both sexes have a characteristic physique. Darlington writes in *Genetics and Man:* "We find men of pronouncedly feminine temperament and physique. We find women of pronouncedly masculine temperament and physique. Such men and women are often more interested in their own sex than in the opposite sex."[3]

Many famous and distinguished men have been homosexual: Oscar Wilde, André Gide, Marcel Proust, Walt Whitman, Christopher Marlowe, Michelangelo, Leonardo da Vinci, and several kings of England—to name only a few. The life histories of these famous men illustrate some of the unusual relationships with parents that are probably among the important causes of homosexuality.

In André Gide's autobiographical novel *If It Die (Si le grain ne meurt*) his mother is presented as gentle and musical and devoted to him. Gide feared and venerated his father, who was professor of law at the Sorbonne. His father "spent most of the day shut up in a vast and rather dark study, into which I was only allowed when he expressly invited me." Gide says of his father's room: "I went into it as into a temple; the bookcase arose out of the gloom like a tabernacle." [4] Gide was an only child and his father died when he was eleven.

Marcel Proust also had a warm, tender-hearted mother and a rather distant father. The personality of Proust's mother can be seen in the mother of the narrator in *Remembrance of Things Past (A la recherche du temps perdu)*. André Maurois writes:

> The tragedy that resulted for Marcel from his discovery of the great world and of himself is to be explained in terms of the brutal contrast between a reality that was harsh and not seldom base and the life he had known in the midst of his own people where he had been sheltered by the goodness of his mother and his grandmother, by their nobility of mind and by their moral principles. These two women seem to have adored and spoiled the delicate child whose temperament so much resembled their own. His father was a more worldly, remote and stern figure who would have liked to see his gifted but over-indulged son submitted to a more stringent discipline. [5]

Study after study has pointed in the same direction, producing a pile of evidence suggesting that childhood experiences are a cause of homosexuality. Irving Bieber, a psychoanalytically trained psychiatrist, found that the mothers of homosexuals often formed binding, intimate relationships with their sons, favoring the son who became homosexual over the other children and sometimes over the husband. [6] The mother would spend an enormous amount of time with him, exchanging confidences, discouraging masculine interests, and interfering with relationships with girls. The mothers were themselves puritanical if not sexually frigid. The fathers were usually emotionally detached or hostile, or openly favored the other children.

However, homosexuality may be caused in a variety of ways. Studies of homosexuals who are not neurotic or under psychiatric treatment do not so strongly suggest overprotective or emotional mothering as a cause of homosexuality. Dr. Eva Bene, a London psychologist, found that homosexuals expressed far more hostility toward their fathers than did heterosexual men, but they also expressed more hostility and less affection toward their mothers. [7]

This suggests that homosexuals are more attached to their mothers than their fathers, not because they have stronger relationships with their mothers than do heterosexuals, but because they have poorer relationships with their fathers. The fathers of homosexuals may themselves wish to be mothered and so be in competition with their sons. This would be a sort of reverse Oedipus complex—the father jealous of the son's relationship with the mother, instead of vice versa. As a result, the son's relationship with the mother is disturbed because of the son's fear of displeasing his father.

The classic Freudian theory of male homosexuality is still valuable and consistent in a general way with many of these observations. Freud suggested that homosexuals have a deep fear of heterosexuality, which develops in childhood as a result of the child's conflicting feelings toward parents. Some men who idolize their mothers are impotent with women of their own class but are able to have sexual relations with prostitutes. Women of the mother's social class must be kept pure and so are forbidden. Homosexuals have gone one stage further and are sexually unresponsive to all women and are able only to respond to their own sex.

The causes of female homosexuality—called lesbianism after the island of Lesbos where the poetess Sappho surrounded herself with female admirers in the fifth century B.C.—are even more of a mystery than the causes of male homosexuality. There has been little interest in lesbianism compared with the quantity of research into male homosexuality. This is undoubtedly because of a taboo on the discussion of the subject that has operated in the past, together with the fact that most research on homosexuality has been done by men who have neglected lesbianism. The taboo on lesbianism in literature was active in England as late as 1928, when Radclyffe Hall's romantic novel *The Well of Loneliness* was withdrawn from circulation at the request of the home secretary. Shortly afterward a magistrate declared the novel obscene and ordered copies of it to be destroyed.

Lesbians have no distinguishing physical or biological features. They menstruate normally and are capable of having babies. The stereotype butch woman with masculine appearance and the ultrafeminine type are probably no more common among lesbians than among women in general.

Doctors at St. Thomas's and Guy's hospitals in London have studied forty-two lesbians in the hope of finding some physical difference between lesbians and heterosexual women. They gave the lesbians every known physical and medical test. They measured nine hormones in their urine and examined and measured every detail of their bodies. They could find virtually no difference between the lesbians and a comparison group of heterosexual women. They concluded that "it is absolutely clear that there is no such thing as a lesbian physique." However, they did find from psychological tests that the lesbian women were more prone to anxiety and tension and less sociable than heterosexual women. Some of these psychological differences might be caused by the strain of having a way of life that is not socially sanctioned. The strain did show in the faces of these women because the doctors remarked (in an article in the learned journal *Nature,* July, 1972) how most of the women looked older than their real age, although this was not a feature that could be measured scientifically.

Dr. Alfred C. Kinsey found in his famous study of *Sexual Behavior in the Human Female* that up to 13 percent of females have some homosexual experience, mostly shortlived. However, some 4 percent of single women could be called practicing lesbians. Kinsey found that women's homosexual experiences were much more likely to be confined to one partner than are the homosexual experiences of men.[8] Lesbian relationships seem to arise most often from strong friendships or protracted romantic attachments. Lesbians are seldom promiscuous and do not go in for one-night stands as homosexual men frequently do. Many women with lesbian inclinations marry, although they probably tend to be frigid and, if they do not learn to enjoy heterosexual relations, may always be swept off their feet by a passionate woman friend late in life.

Important causes of lesbianism, like male homosexuality, may lie in childhood experiences. Dr. F. E. Kenyon, a psychiatrist, found that the early emotional life of lesbian women was much more disturbed than that of a comparison group of heterosexual women. The lesbians studied by Kenyon were more likely to have had poor relationships with their mothers, who were more likely to have had mental disturbances or to have died. They were also more likely to have had disturbed relationships with their fathers, and their parents were more likely to have been separated or divorced.

Fewer lesbians in the study remembered that they had a happy childhood. Forty percent of them could remember a particularly traumatic sexual advance from a man, whereas only about 25 percent of heterosexual women had had that kind of traumatic sexual experience. Nevertheless, more than half the lesbians had experience of heterosexual intercourse and a quarter of them wanted to become exclusively heterosexual. The lesbians did not so often regard themselves as fully feminine and many more of them had worked in the uniformed women's services.[9]

Another study of female homosexuals in London, made by Dr. Eva Bene, suggests that the cause of female homosexuality may lie in a defective relationship with the father rather than the mother. Dr. Bene's findings came as a surprise to many psychoanalysts, who since Freud have looked for defects in the mother-child relationship as the cause of both female and male homosexuality. Dr. Bene found that lesbians were more often hostile to their fathers and afraid of them than were married women, and they more often felt that their fathers were weak and incompetent.[10]

Studies in the United States have also found that unstable family backgrounds are an important contributing factor to homosexuality in girls. Dr. Malvina W. Kremer of New York University School of Medicine and Dr. Alfred H. Rifkin of New York Medical College studied twenty-five lesbians between the ages of twelve and seventeen in New York City. The girls grew up in families that were unstable, men came and went, and they never had a reliable father figure in their lives. Their security came entirely from their mothers. This again suggests that girls need a father figure to whom they can relate successfully if they are to have an enjoyable sexual relationship with men later in life.[11] But there is still the possibility that stress on the mothers or directly on the girls themselves may have produced some subtle alteration in body function through hormones.

Homosexuality in men and women might be caused by some difference in body chemistry that affects the mind but not the physique. It is possible that there is a larger variation in the quantity of the male hormone testosterone in the blood of male homosexuals than in that of heterosexuals. Men with low quantities of testosterone in their blood are possibly more likely to be homosexual, but it is also possible that a homosexual pattern of life actually changes hormone levels in the blood. It is well known that people's hormones are affected by their state of mind. Messages from the brain acting via the pituitary gland can alter the hormone balance of the body. For example, a woman who is depressed or shocked may not have her normal monthly periods.

In monkeys the quantity of testosterone in the blood reflects a monkey's status in the colony. Dr. Irwin Bernstein at Yerkes Regional Primate Research Center in Atlanta, Georgia, has found that a rhesus monkey who is boss of a colony tends to have higher levels of testosterone than monkeys lower in the hierarchy. And the boss monkeys are not always the physically fittest specimens. To be boss in a rhesus monkey colony depends as much on what friends a monkey has—which other monkeys will give support—as on how strong a monkey is. Bernstein proved the relationship by removing some of the boss monkey's friends so that he could no longer maintain his status. A coup followed in the colony and the leader's testosterone plummeted as another group of monkeys took over. The amount of testosterone in the blood of the new leader rose above what it was before. Similar changes in testosterone level occurred when leader monkeys were transferred to another group that did not recognize their leadership.[12]

It seems possible that exposure of the growing embryo within the womb to excessive quantities of hormones from the mother might be another cause of homosexuality. The excessive hormones might originate within the mother's own body as a result of the action of stress on the adrenal gland or of psychological factors on the pituitary gland, or the hormones might even originate in particular foods. Exposure at one stage of pregnancy or in one way might produce the transsexual person, while exposure in another way or at another time in pregnancy might turn the growing baby into a homosexual.

If homosexuality is sometimes or partly caused by hormones in the womb, there would be little possibility of changing the inclinations of homosexuals by injections of hormones later in life: experiments with animals show that once the brain has developed sexually it cannot be reversed. It has long been known that homosexuality in both men and women does not respond to treatment with hormones. Indeed, it is this observation that has always encouraged doctors to look for the causes of homosexuality in early life.

A recent treatment for sexual disorders is the synthetic hormone cyproterone acetate, which acts as a sexual tranquillizer by counteracting the effect of testosterone. Men with excessive sexual appetites who are given the drug are able to control their appetites and keep them within normal bounds.

Trials in Britain and Germany show that sexually aggressive men who have been before the courts have frequently improved when given the drug, and sadomasochists who have taken it have found their fantasies less compelling. One English university graduate who wanted intercourse twenty times a week—to an extent that he said it was interfering with his social life—was satisfied with twice-weekly intercourse after taking the drug. Some doctors hoped that the drug might hold out a cure for homosexuality, but they were disappointed. The drug has the same effect on the homosexual sex drive as on the heterosexual drive. It damps down the sex drive but does not alter its direction.

The environmental theory of the cause of homosexuality is not incompatible with the hormone theory. Even if special exposure to hormones in the womb is proved to be a cause of homosexuality, there must be large numbers of people whose fate is not finally decided in the womb and will still be influenced one way or the other by their social or family experiences.

However, if abnormal exposure to hormones in the womb is a cause of homosexuality, then we must face the alarming possibility that some people might take steps to prevent homosexuality by persuading pregnant mothers to have injections of sex hormones. Technically there is no reason why the procedure could not be applied now by many doctors if there were a demand for it.

First it would be necessary to determine the sex of the fetus by an operation known as amniocentesis. This is done by removing some of the liquid surrounding the fetus with a long needle that pierces the womb. Then the chromosomes in the cells present in the liquid must be examined to discover the sex of the fetus. Once the sex of the fetus is known, it could be "reinforced" at about the fourth or fifth month with injections of the appropriate hormone.

The results for society as a whole of the widespread use of such methods of channeling and exaggerating the differences between the sexes are difficult to imagine. Homosexuals have always boasted of the large numbers of creative people who are homosexual. Would these people have been equally creative if they were heterosexual and had not gone through the torment of adjustment in adolescence that so many homosexuals experience? It is impossible to say. But society would surely be less tolerant of deviations and the arts less varied once a program of sexual normalization began.

In Hitler's Germany, homosexuals risked being sent to the gas chambers. Should such a society arise again, the possibility of sex-reinforcement treatment of the fetus using hormones is not unthinkable. The result might be an even more aggressive class of warrior males and women subjected to even more submissive and humiliating roles. Such treatment would override any natural controlling forces that may exist, such as those discovered by Dr. John Calhoun in his experimental mouse universe. If an analogy with Dr. Calhoun's mouse universe is valid, then as aggression increases in human society, the birth rate will fall and babies may be less aggressive and less extremely masculine or feminine. In an open society, as opposed to the closed mouse universe, the hormonal response of the mother to her environment may act as a regulator controlling the aggressiveness and sexuality of future generations. If this is so, then any attempt to interfere could have explosive consequences.

It would be a mistake to pursue the analogy with animals too far. Human beings are unique in the number of factors that can combine and contrive to distort sexual behavior. Prolonged childhood, during which we are emotionally dependent upon parents, and appearance of the sex drive long before it can be easily satisfied influence men and women to seek homosexual relationships.

Biologically the homosexual relationship remains a puzzle. Homosexuals obviously do not reproduce themselves as effectively as heterosexuals and so there must be an evolutionary selection against homosexuality. How, then, can we explain the large proportion of homosexuals in the population? They are far too numerous to be constantly arising only from genetic mutation and genetic recombination. This consideration alone must reinforce the importance of looking further for the causes of homosexuality in childhood and adolescent experiences.

Belief that homosexuality is inherited encourages the belief that it is an unalterable condition. Nothing could be further from the truth. Many men who are homosexual as teen-agers and in their early twenties settle down to normal marriage and a happy heterosexual sex life later. This is one of the most important conclusions to come from Dr. A. C. Kinsey's investigations of the *Sexual Behavior of the Human Male*. Kinsey also found that about 10 percent of younger married men had had homosexual experience since their marriages and that other men had changed from an exclusively heterosexual to an exclusively homosexual way of life. Among women, homosexuality appears even more likely to occupy only a short phase in life, lasting perhaps no more than a few years.

Only a relatively small minority of homosexuals want to be "cured." The most vocal gay liberation groups strongly reject the idea of treating homosexuality as if it were a disease. They campaign for the right of a person to be free to love others in his or her own way. And they are interested in helping homosexuals to stop feeling guilty about being gay. Homosexuals, like women and blacks, have been persecuted and maligned in the past.

Hereditarian science has reflected the popular view and so has aided and abetted the political moves against homosexuals. It has condemned homosexuals, with criminals, as the inheritors of "bad"

genes. The dilemma of the homosexual is the same as that of other
minorities who have been victims of the superman cult in our society.
He-men such as John Wayne or Clark Kent, the original Superman,
have not just typified an ideal of virility, they have left the homosexual
playing the role of funny man or dude. But it is strange that no major
film has yet been made (apart perhaps from Warhol's *Lonesome Cow-
boy*) that tells the truth about homosexuality on the prairies of the Wild
West, where women were hard to come by and men apparently
learned how to do without.

There is no conclusive scientific evidence to show that homosexuals of either sex are biologically any different from heterosexual men
and women. Studies made by Franz Kallman of identical homosexual
twins in New York in 1952 are still quoted as evidence that homosexuality is inherited. Kallman's homosexual twins, many of whom were
obtained with the collaboration of the New York City and New York
State departments of correction, were mostly criminal or severely abnormal in other ways that make it impossible to generalize from his
findings. Furthermore, most of his twins were raised not separately but
within the same family, where they were subject to the same environmental influences. This work has simply served to confirm popular
prejudice and bolster the hereditarian view of society.[13]

The balance of evidence suggests that homosexuals learn, albeit
unconsciously, the sexual preferences they have. They are not being
driven by instinct because they may—at least sometimes—choose to
change and are often able to do so gradually without any professional
help. Many other homosexuals have no wish to change and settle
down permanently into a homosexual way of life, often with one partner. There is hope, too, for those homosexuals who do wish to change
but cannot do it alone—especially if they are young and have limited
homosexual experience. By means of psychotherapy a homosexual's
fears of the opposite sex may sometimes be gradually removed and
confidence built up until he or she is able to begin a heterosexual relationship. This treatment is often long and difficult and the outcome uncertain, but there is no doubt that cure is possible. Other male homosexuals who seek to change their life have been successfully treated by
behavior therapy. In this technique the patient is "punished" with
mild electric shocks when he chooses to look at pictures of men and
rewarded by withholding the shocks when he chooses to look at pictures of women. Using this method a homosexual may gradually learn
to alter his fantasies and develop an interest in the opposite sex—but it

must be done in such a way that fear of women is removed while inhibition towards men develops.

What must surely be the most enjoyable method of treatment for homosexuality has been called seduction therapy by D. J. West, a lecturer in criminology in Cambridge, England, who is an authority on homosexuality. Dr. West describes the case of an attractive young woman who came to see him offering her services as a volunteer to help male homosexuals overcome their fears. Her boyfriend had been a homosexual, and by persistence she had managed to laugh away his fears until he had overcome his inhibitions and was able to enjoy intercourse. Once she had freed him of his fears in this way, he left her and went off with another woman. Foreseeing further disappointments, Dr. West advised her to find a normal man.[14]

CHAPTER 7

Sex in Society

"Is it a boy or a girl?" is the first question people ask when their baby is born. It seems more important to know this than to know if it is healthy or if it has been harmed by the delivery. Once the baby's sex is known, the process of cultural brainwashing may safely begin. Many people still dress girls in pink and boys in blue so that from the beginning there can be no doubt about their sex so far as the rest of the world is concerned. Noticing the color of the baby's clothes, friends and relatives then find their cue for making appropriate remarks such as "What a fine fellow" or "What a pretty little thing." From the beginning the baby is subjected to assumptions about itself and its nature based on the simple observation of its sex.

Mothers treat newborn male and female babies differently. In one study, made by psychologist H. A. Moss, it was discovered that male babies slept less than females and were more irritable and so required more comforting.[1] Other differences between the sexes have been found from birth. Baby girls are more sensitive to touch and pain and can hear better than baby boys. Baby boys, however, are able to see better. Baby girls at twelve weeks will spend longer staring at photographs of faces than at geometric figures, whereas boys pay equal attention to both, although in their early school years, boys give more attention to geometric shapes. Similar differences appear to exist in later life when men, as Kinsey observed, are more easily aroused by erotic pictures whereas women are more easily aroused by feelings of touch. Other observations also suggest that there may be differences between the way in which the brains of men and women function. It has been suggested that the right half of the brain functions differently in the two sexes.

The right side of the brain is used more than the left side to control movement in space and to interpret perception, as opposed to language, which is controlled by the left side of the brain. At least, this is the most usual arrangement found in right-handed people; in left-handed people the division of function may be more blurred. When different sets of numbers are repeated at the same time into each ear, most people are able to repeat the numbers fed into the right ear more accurately. The numbers fed into the *right* ear are processed on the *left* side of the brain, which is better at the job. On the other hand, if different musical tunes are fed into right and left ears, those fed into the left ear and processed on the right side of the brain are best recalled.

Psychologists A. W. H. Buffery and J. A. Gray have suggested that girls develop language ability earlier because the left side of their brain matures earlier. They say that this is why most boys do not learn to use the left side of their brains as fully as girls. They suggest that boys use this extra brain capacity for interpreting movements in space, which explains the common male superiority in controlling movement.[2] However, there is a large element of speculation in this theory. Why, for example, should females be superior in language because the brainwork is concentrated on one side of the brain and males be superior in movement because the brainwork is shared between both sides? It seems as if the theory has it both ways. It is just as likely that differences in the functioning of the brain in the two sexes develop through cultural training. By talking more to their mothers girls develop abilities that are controlled by the left side of the brain, while boys develop their control of movement through having more practice and encouragement in it.

Tests of some intellectual abilities show interesting differences between men and women. Girls tend to have higher IQ scores up to the age of about six and boys tend to have higher scores during puberty. Girls are especially good with words. They learn to speak and read sooner than boys and are on the average more fluent with words and able to use longer sentences. Throughout their lives girls remain more fluent with words and better at grammar and spelling, but boys tend to catch up eventually. In their teens boys show a greater than average ability with numbers, while girls are better at music and art.

However, gifted girls with high IQs often do not live up to their potential either in schoolwork or in their jobs. They appear to be holding themselves back. In later life there is some correlation between a

man's job and his IQ, but with women the correlation is virtually
nonexistent. One study of gifted children followed through to adult-
hood found a close relationship between a man's job and his IQ but
virtually no relationship for women, although both started in the same
range of high IQ as gifted children. Two thirds of those women who
as adults had IQs of 170 or over—in the genius range—were house-
wives or office workers. The women in this study also showed on
average a greater drop in IQ as adolescents and young adults than did
the men.[3]

Boys seem to be able to convert IQ into achievement, but girls find
it much more difficult. This difficulty begins at puberty, when pressure
for them to adopt their expected gender role is most intense. Girls
perhaps fear that if they do well academically they will be less attractive to boys. This may lead them to pretend to be less intelligent than
boys, and ultimately the pretense may become reality, with a decline
in IQ. This again shows that IQ is not a quantity fixed at birth but is
dependent upon the environment. Ability, as measured in IQ tests, can
also decline in men after the school years when they get boring jobs
and gradually lose interest in words, numbers, and ideas.

The differences in intellectual ability between the sexes have been
explained by some as being caused by heredity and by others as being
caused by environment. Environmental theories of differences in intellectual abilities are generally more convincing. Evidence suggests that
the parent of opposite sex may be a crucial factor in the development
of high intellectual ability for both boys and girls. For example, psychologist David Levy found that boys who were overprotected by their
mothers and overdependent on them developed a feminine style of intellectual ability.[4] These boys had greater verbal skills and poorer analytical ability than the average boy. On the other hand, women with
unusually high analytical ability in psychological tests have been
found to identify more closely with their fathers. And women mathe-
maticians are found to have particularly strong attachments to their fathers.

Gender roles vary in different families and in different societies. The
terms *male* and *female* are constant in meaning, but the concept of
what is masculine or feminine varies. Among the Manus in New
Guinea the care of babies is associated with the masculine gender role,
and when anthropologist Margaret Mead presented Manus children
with dolls for the first time it was the boys who showed most interest
in them and played with them. In Western society, the popular view

seems to be that differences in gender roles reflect innate and inevitable differences between the sexes.

This belief that masculine and feminine gender roles are innate stems from an unquestioning acceptance of the way in which our society is organized. It is not possible for fathers to be present in the home for most of the day. This situation is rationalized by the belief that the woman's place is in the home. Because the woman is in the home, she then assumes the service duties associated with the home. Ann Oakley puts it cogently in her book *Sex, Gender and Society:*

> The asymmetrical structure of the family—father at work, mother at home—allows a connection to be made between such diverse activities as the feeding of tiny babies, the cleaning of houses, and the washing of dirty socks. In reality, while childbearing is a biological function, and therefore female, domestic work is a social/economic one, and therefore sexually neuter; but where both are in practice feminine, the biological role of motherhood takes on a whole aura of domesticity and cultural femininity. The lines are tied between the act of giving birth and the act of cleaning the house, and the status of women as a group is colored by these secondary cultural consequences of the primary biological specialization. From that point on, it is not biology that determines the role of women, but domesticity.[5]

The domestic roles carry over into the job market, where the better jobs commonly available to women are in the paradomestic service professions of nurse, secretary, or teacher. Few women have jobs as foremen, managers, or executives. The majority of women are employed in repetitive factory work that employers often justify on the grounds that it is temperamentally more suited to women. Males command the majority of jobs that carry high prestige and high income. The hours women work and the jobs they can do are limited by law in many countries, but these limitations often appear to be designed to protect male interests as much as to protect women from exploitation. For example, in Ohio women are legally barred from work in small factories (employing fourteen people or less) that might require them to lift more than fifteen pounds in weight—the weight a baby reaches in the first few months of life. Similar restrictions were repealed in California in 1971. The Ohio law has not yet been challenged, but it is doubtful if it would withstand appeal.

Women who seek a career are caught in a double-bind situation: they can't win. In the United States a study of femininity and success made by Harvard psychologist Matina Horner, who is also president of Radcliffe College, shows that women actively fear success.[6] She

found that 65 percent of women whom she asked to write about a successful woman associated success in their own sex with depression,
illness, and sometimes death. In the same test 90 percent of men associated success with happiness and prosperity. She also found that the
greater a woman's fear of competition with men, the less she
achieved. It appears to be fear of the consequences of success, rather
than innate preference or limited ability, that drives women to seek
jobs in traditional roles. What is more, this fear is justified. Men do not
think of the stereotypical successful women as attractive. Male law
students tested by Matina Horner described successful women as unat-
tractive, unfeminine, and overaggressive. Despite superficial changes,
we are still light years away from a unisex society, let alone a society
that gives women modest opportunities to compete on equal terms.

We use the word *sexism* to describe the prejudice and obstruction
women experience at the hands of men. Sexism, like racism, is based
on a biological genetic difference that has become institutionalized.
Discrimination on the basis of sex or color is easy to effect because
these are physical differences that a person cannot change. Sociologist
Helen Hacker has made a detailed comparison of the parallels between
sexism and racism.[7] She points out that black people are said to have a
lesser range of intelligence, with fewer geniuses among their number,
and so are women. One reason given for this is that black people are
supposed to have smaller and less convoluted brains than white men
have—the same has been said of women. Black people, according to
popular prejudice, are freer in their instinctual gratifications: they are
more primitive, childlike, irresponsible, inconsistent, and emotionally
unstable. Women are popularly believed to have these faults, too.
Prejudice has it that black people are inferior and that women are the
weaker sex—and "weaker" often seems to imply more than just lack
of physical strength. These are the prejudicial labels that women and
negroes must contend with, says Ms. Hacker.

Ms. Hacker points out that men rationalize the status of women—
as they may rationalize the status of negroes—by saying that women
are contented in their role and cause less trouble when they are kept in
their place. And the conventional place for the woman is in the home.
She also points out that women are forced to use flattery to gain their
ends and black people are forced to use deference. Women often ac-
commodate to men's views with a show of ignorance or helplessness,
concealing their real feelings, and negroes are often forced to adopt
the same tactics. The result of these adaptations to the white *man's*

domination are the stereotypes that Ms. Hacker describes of the help-less woman and the ignorant negro who nevertheless sometimes outwit the white menfolk. Women and negroes, each in their own way, are put in a position where they cannot win: if they stick up for themselves as individuals with rights, they are considered to be uppity, and if they use some guile to gain their ends because there is no other way, they are seen as wily or bewitching, and if they are compliant, they are as-sumed to be happy with their lot.

Sexism, like racism, was taken to extremes by the Nazis in Ger-many in the period between the 1930s and the end of the Second World War. Their persecution of women, although the most savage in recent history, has passed almost unnoticed except by feminists such as Kate Millett, author of *Sexual Politics*. Women's organizations were infiltrated by Nazis and taken over by the Nazi party. Once the opposi-tion was stifled, a policy was enforced of taking women out of the pro-fessions and putting them back into the home or into low-paid occupa-tions. Women were forced into "sacred motherhood" when contraceptives were made illegal. In December, 1934, Dr. Gerhardt Wagner, leader of the medical profession and of the German medical delegation to the Nazi party meeting of 1935, said, "We will strangle higher education for women." [8] Professional women were fired or forced to resign by legislation against "double-income families." The only alternative was some humble job in a service role. Hitler justified this policy by saying that it was woman's nature to do these things. He is quoted in the Nazi Woman's handbook as saying:

> We do not find it right when the woman presses into the world of man. Rather we find it natural when these two worlds remain separate. To one belongs the power of feeling, the power of soul . . . to the other belongs the strength of vision, the strength of hardness. . . . The man upholds the nation as the woman upholds the family. The equal rights of woman consist in the fact that in the realm of life determined for her by nature she experiences the high esteem which is her due. [9]

To help create the Nazi superman, women were prescribed a slave role from which it was virtually impossible to escape.

Hitler was not the originator of these ideas. Such theories were commonly accepted at that time, even by scientists—at least in Ger-many. Dr. Fritz Lenz, professor of racial hygiene at the University of Munich, wrote in the popular textbook *Human Heredity:* "Each sex has its own peculiar tasks to fulfill in the life of the race, and must be fitted for these tasks by the inheritance of particular bodily and mental characteristics.'' [10] And this is how he saw the differences between men and women:

> A woman wishes, above all, to be regarded as beautiful and desirable, whereas a man wants to be regarded as a hero and as a person who gets things done. Man has more courage than woman in attack, whereas woman shows more valiancy in suffering. Since women are selected by nature mainly for the breeding of children and for the allurement of men, their interests are dependent upon those of men and of children, and are directed towards persons rather than towards things. Owing to the particular nature of her part in life, woman is endowed with more imaginative insight, more empathy, than man. She can readily put herself in another's place, she lives more for others, her main motive being her love for husband and children—and her desire to foster illusions in her husband's mind. [11]

Similar sexist ideas are not difficult to find in currently popular scientific writing, for example in the writings of C. D. Darlington. His analysis of the origins of the differences between men and women begins with reference to fish. He writes in *Genetics and Man:*

> The sexes [in different species of animals] may be alike or widely divergent. In certain fishes the male attaches itself in infancy to the belly of the female and there, incapable of independent life, it continues without further growth or movement, a parasite for the rest of its existence. The divergence of the sexes in man is less serious but still physically and mentally profound. [12]

To Darlington men and women are no less different genetically than two related species. His analysis continues into the social and political sphere and gives scientific backing to the idea that the sexes are basically inevitably unequal.

> How absurd it is for us to speak of the two sexes as being equal! Clearly they are not. They overlap in particular respects. But taken as a whole, they are different. Each has its value, a value best appreciated by the other, a value the result of long selection and adaptation. Just as with two races and two classes, equality can only be in relation to some particular scale, some particular terms of reference. [13]

The achievements of women are attributed by Darlington to ''the positively homosexual type of woman'' who ''has become by her own faculties and by her own choice, the mouthpiece of the less articulate and feminine part of her sex.'' He says, ''She [the positive female homosexual] is notably masculine in her type of intelligence yet she is responsible for what is happily called feminism.'' [14] These remarks would not be of such interest if they had not been made by an Oxford professor in a major work on the biology of man. Again, they put women in a position where they cannot win. If women compete with men they are presumed to be homosexual, and if they do not they are "unequal," if not actually inferior. It would be difficult to find a better example of sexism. These views totally ignore the social context of men and women, as if their environment were no more complicated than a fishbowl. Kate Millett recognizes this scientific sexism. She says:

> One of the most unfortunate aspects of civilization is the extent to which learning and scientific interest are so deeply affected by the culture in which such study is done. A Nazi state invents its own Nazi social investigation; a racist state can formulate a racist science to sanction its most passionate hatreds. While the social sciences in America are just now being purged of a racist bias indulged with considerable freedom over many decades, a strong "sexist" bias, the product of several decades of reaction, still pervades such areas of study . . . the most formidable task of reactionary opinion was to blur or disguise distinctions in status while re-emphasizing sexual differences in personality by implying that they are innate rather than cultural.[15]

Women have been given the same shoddy deal by science as black men, criminals, and those who suffer from mental illness or tuberculosis. Rationalizations of woman's inferior role by pseudobiological and genetic arguments have been universal in Western countries, if not throughout the world.

The strength of purely biological influences on the roles of men and women in society is difficult to estimate. At present there are still so many social and legal ways in which women are repressed that biology is of secondary importance. It is possible that the social roles of men and women are influenced by differences in sex hormones in their bodies that make men more competitive and women relatively passive. But as long as women are legally and socially restricted it is impossible to attempt to evaluate the importance of any biological influences apart from the basic fact that only women can bear children and breast-feed them.

The major causes of the different roles of men and women in our society have in reality nothing directly to do with biology or genetics but are almost wholly social and economic. There are very few jobs that cannot be done as well by women—and indeed are done by women in other cultures. In the past nature itself has been the oppressor of women. Now that women's role in the bearing and feeding of children has been lessened by the contraceptive pill and the baby bottle, there is the possibility of a new treaty between the sexes with more flexible ways of bringing up children. In theory there seems to be no reason why men should not spend more time at home and women go out to work, if they want to. Women are prevented by our sexist society from doing much that is within their powers. We are all losers as a result.

Sexism is as much a threat to individual freedom as racism. But sexism is in some ways more insidious. It so permeates our lives that it is more difficult to recognize and come to terms with. Sexual stereotypes are constantly bombarding us on television and in literature, and the same stereotypes have been adopted by hereditarian science. Our lives are built on an assumption that men and women are innately different and that labor should be divided in a prescribed way between the sexes. Men are prisoners of their work and women are prisoners in the home, while neither role alone can be truly satisfying. The ideal solution is provided, perhaps, when a man and woman can share a job between them—as when a family runs a small business. Another solution is for both to work part-time. Whatever the practical solution, a man can grow in feeling and understanding through being more closely involved in bringing up his children, and a woman can bring more back to the family when she maintains real links with the outside world.

If only a few men and women could adapt to less restricted sex roles it could do much to combat the more insidious effects of sexism. Among these is the glorification of aggression and violence as the superlative power of men. Girls are molded into service roles while boys are encouraged to play at superman. The encouragement of such sexist fantasies can only further divide men and women and increase the violence in our society. Rape, wife-beating, beating up homosexuals, and even baby-battering are among the evil fruits of the predominantly male cult of violence.

This might begin to change if we did more to teach boys a caring role and encouraged girls to become more creative. We could begin in quite small ways by suggesting, for example, that boys play with dolls, which are the first models a child has for practicing care. Little boys can also be encouraged to play at nurses, and girls at doctors, so that both sexes at an early age learn to understand the different types of responsibility involved in care. More schools should give boys an opportunity to learn cooking and sewing, and girls an opportunity to learn carpentry and metalwork. It should not be assumed that men and women are automatically suited for the roles they assume in life. Change is possible: there is nothing biologically inevitable about the present roles and status of men and women. And so the message is reject sexist propaganda, forget the sexual stereotypes, aim to discover who you really want to be, and negotiate with your mate a personal compromise that works for you.

CRIME

Scholars and scientists who study crime have to enter a foreign culture and, like early travelers to a foreign land, have sometimes returned with the most extraordinary travelers' tales. Among the mythical monsters of crime that scientists have reported are the born criminal with protruding ears and a receding chin, the identical twin who, long separated from his brother, commits the same copybook crime at the same time hundreds of miles away, and the "Y-factor" criminal who is driven by his unlucky heredity to a life of destruction. These are all pseudo-scientific myths, but scientists themselves have encouraged belief in them.

Locked into their scholarly lives, biologists and psychologists have often been puzzled by the life and culture of criminals. They have asked: Why is one man good and another bad? Where does our sense of right and wrong originate? And they have looked to heredity for the answer. But contrary to hereditarian teaching, it has never been demonstrated scientifically that people become criminals as a result of inevitable hereditary processes. Many criminals learn to go straight and many honest people are corrupted by circumstances.

CHAPTER 8

The Criminal Instinct: Born or Bred?

One day in about 1870, Cesare Lombroso, the first modern theorist of crime, was examining the skull of the famous Italian brigand Vihella. He had a "flash of inspiration," which he later described like this:

> At the sight of that skull, I seemed to see all of a sudden, lighted up as a vast plain under a flaming sky, the problem of the nature of the criminal—an atavistic being who reproduces in his person the ferocious instincts of primitive humanity and the inferior animals. Thus were explained anatomically the enormous jaws, high cheek bones, prominent superciliary arches, solitary lines in the palms, extreme size of the orbits, handle-shaped or sensile ears found in criminals, savages and apes, insensibility to pain, extremely acute sight, tattooing, excessive idleness, love of orgies, and the irresistible craving for evil for its own sake, the desire not only to extinguish life in the victim, but to mutilate the corpse, tear its flesh and drink its blood.[1]

Lombroso, who was a doctor, then set out to gather evidence to support his theory by taking measurements on four hundred Italian prisoners and comparing them with soldiers. He found that 43 percent of criminals had five or more "anomalies" such as abnormal size or shape of head, receding chin, or long arms, whereas none of the soldiers had as many as five of these anomalies and only 11 percent had as many as three. Lombroso overlooked the possibility that the soldiers might have been specially selected for their good health and good looks, and concluded that the existence of these anomalies supported the idea of a "born criminal type." Lombroso suggested that criminals were an evolutionary "throwback" to an earlier form of human or animal life. This suggestion had first been made by Darwin a few years before in his book *The Descent of Man*. Darwin said: "With mankind some of the worst dispositions which occasionally without any assignable cause make their appearance in families, may perhaps be reversions to a savage state, from which we are not removed by many generations." [2]

Lombroso's theory put any person with physical defects or peculiarities under suspicion of having hidden criminal leanings. Included in large numbers among the criminal suspects were the lower classes, who because of their arduous life and poor nutrition were more likely to have physical peculiarities. But the political implications of Lombroso's theory went beyond this. In another investigation of the anatomical peculiarities of "anarchists," i.e., those who were members of an extreme political group, he discovered that up to 40 percent of them had physical "blemishes," as compared with only 12 percent of the ranks of other extremist political movements. Lombroso was linking physical deformity with both crime and the anarchist political movement.

The idea that criminals can be recognized by stigmata—whether these are found in the chromosomes, the facial features, or the brain—goes back at least to biblical times. Cain carried marks that were said to betray his criminal nature. Perhaps it is comforting for the rest of us who are law-abiding to think of the criminal and the delinquent as people entirely apart—completely separated by physical differences. This would explain the continuing popularity of such theories.

However, Lombroso's observations have never stood up to careful testing. When in 1913 Dr. Charles Goring, a medical criminologist, carefully compared three thousand English prisoners and nonprisoners, including Oxford and Cambridge undergraduates, he was scarcely able to establish any significant differences. The prisoners were found to be slightly shorter and to weigh less. These were almost certainly only signs of poorer nutrition either in early life or later in prison. Goring concluded that "there is no such thing as the criminal type." [3]

However, the idea persisted, and in 1939 Ernest Hooton, a Harvard anthropologist, published his three-volume work *The American Criminal*. Over a period of twelve years, Hooton had measured ten thousand criminals and compared them with a smaller control group. His conclusions had a familiar ring about them. He found that criminals were "organically inferior" and "low grade human organisms." He wrote: "The elimination of crime can only be effected by the extirpation of the physically, mentally, and morally unfit; or by their complete segregation in a socially aseptic environment.'' [4]

Hooton never explained on what grounds he considered his indicators of criminality—such as narrow jaws, compressed faces, and low, sloping foreheads—to be signs of inferiority. He included among these signs tattooing, which is common among prisoners, who often do it out of boredom and to be like their friends. But it is difficult to see how a tattoo can indicate anything more than the desire to be tattooed and the existence of an environment that looks favorably upon it. Hooton's massive work was unconvincing for other reasons. He did not make any special attempt to find a group of men who would provide a fair comparison with the prisoners. The men he compared them with included hospital patients, college students, the patrons of a bathing beach, and others who happened to be available. As it turned out, he found that a group of Nashville firemen differed more from a group of Boston men than either did from the prisoners. Hooton appeared to be convinced from the outset that the prisoners must be inferior because they were in prison.

The idea that there is something inherently different in the physical makeup of criminals has frequently recurred. The latest unproven theory is that people with certain types of fingerprints are more likely to be criminal than people with other types of fingerprints. If there had been any possible practical use for such observations, the police would have been on to it long ago. All such observations, which are usually merely suggestive, simply reinforce the mistaken idea that criminals are a race apart.

Another suggestion of this type made by two American psychiatrists from the University of Kansas is that criminals suffer from a ''Quasimodo complex.'' Quasimodo, a character in Victor Hugo's *The Hunchback of Notre Dame,* became a recluse as a result of his deformity and turned to antisocial behavior. Dr. F. W. Masters and Dr. D. C. Greaves examined photographs of over eleven thousand murderers, rapists, sex deviants, prostitutes, and suicide victims in five American cities and found that 60 percent of these people were deformed in some way that could be corrected by plastic surgery. This compared with a figure of 2 percent of the general public. They claimed that protruding ears (52 percent) and receding chins (18 percent) were the commonest features of criminals. Ugly noses and acne scars were the main deformities in women.[5] Put at its simplest, the idea behind their study was that ugliness can cause crime.

Whether or not these observations are correct, they cannot be taken as a sign that criminals come from degenerate stock, as has often been suggested by others. The cause of the deformity may be a deprived childhood, which may also have led the person into crime. Alternatively—like both Quasimodo and the original monster of Dr. Frankenstein—the deformed appearance of a person may drive him into social isolation and crime. Protruding ears, the most commonly observed "deformity," may simply be an illusion produced by short prison haircuts.

The best case for the existence of a criminal type has been made by Hans Eysenck in his book *Crime and Personality*. Eysenck believes that the criminal has a different type of nervous system, which is less easily trained to behave in ways acceptable to society. According to his theory, human conscience is a "culmination of a long process of conditioning." [6] He suggests that extroverts are more likely to become criminal because they have inherited a nervous system that is less easily conditioned. According to Eysenck, there is plenty of evidence that criminals are more than normally extroverted and more adaptable and confident in unknown situations. Eysenck bolsters this theory by quoting evidence that criminals on the whole have an "endomorphic" body type (thick-set and muscular), which is typical of extroverts. However, a young lad may have to be strong, well-built, and extroverted to be allowed into a delinquent subculture, or may to some extent develop a stronger physique and more extroverted personality through association with the delinquent subculture. Interesting though the observations are, they prove nothing. Eysenck's theory that criminality is in large measure inherited because the nervous systems of criminals are not easily conditioned, and so do not respond to parental discipline, seems to be simply speculation.

Crime does run in some families. In the past this simple observation has been taken to show that a tendency to commit crimes is inherited. However, it is now recognized by the vast majority of scientists that the simple examination of human pedigrees cannot distinguish between factors in the environment and inheritance in predisposing toward crime. Families have good and bad traditions that are often passed as firmly from one generation to the next as are their genes. The most often quoted examples of criminal families are the Jukes and the Kallikaks, who were first investigated about a hundred years ago. The scientific value of these family pedigree studies is now completely discredited. They would scarcely be worth mentioning were it not that

Professor William Shockley, who won the Nobel Prize for his contributions to the design of the transistor, has tried to revive interest in the tale as part of his campaign to persuade the world that depravity and low intelligence are inherited. One April 23, 1969, Professor Shockley and a few allies wrote a letter to his fellow members of the American National Academy of Sciences:

> We believe that irrefutable evidence continues for the inheritance of genetically controlled, socially maladaptive traits. These findings support the extensive family pedigree studies extending over six generations of the Jukes, Kallikaks, Nams, Ishmaelites and others reported by the Eugenics Record Office of the Carnegie Institute of Washington up to about 1926. . . . The latest FBI report estimates that during the last four years the U.S. homicide rate has increased 33 percent. . . . We fear that ''fatuous beliefs'' in the power of welfare money, unaided by eugenic foresight, may contribute to the decline of human quality for both the black and the white segments of our society and that the fears of genetic deterioration expressed by Jensen . . . are sound and significant.[7]

In the 1870s a prison inspector, R. L. Dugdale, investigated a family in New York State called the Jukes (a made-up name).[8] The family was regarded as having degenerated as a result of heavy inbreeding. More than two thousand members of the Jukes family were traced: all were the descendants of two brothers who married two disreputable sisters in the eighteenth century. Of the descendants, 378 died in infancy, 301 were illegitimate, 366 were paupers, 80 habitual thieves, 171 convicted of other crimes including 10 murders, 175 were prostitutes, and 50 who had venereal disease infected 600 other persons. It has been calculated that between 1800 and 1915 the Jukes cost New York State $2.5 million. Dugdale himself stressed environmental conditions in interpreting this pedigree, but eugenicists have always taken it to support their case.

The Jukes family is always compared with the family of Jonathan Edwards of Connecticut, born in 1703, who by 1900 had at least 1,394 descendants. Of these 15 were presidents of universities, 65 professors in universities, 60 doctors of medicine, 100 clergymen or missionaries, 75 army or navy officers, 60 prominent authors, 130 lawyers (30 of whom became judges), 80 public officers (including 1 vice-president), and 3 senators. At first it was claimed that there was not a single criminal in the Edwards pedigree, but later some were uncovered. The Jukes family was also followed up later, in 1916, and many of the surviving descendants were then found to be good citizens. This improvement was attributed to an infusion of new blood.

The story of the Kallikaks is similar to that of the Jukes and shows how such research into pedigrees can become nothing more than a display of moral virtue. It has more in common with fairy tales or horror stories than with science.

In the early 1900s, Dr. H. H. Goddard, an authority on mental defect, became interested in two distantly related families in New Jersey. One branch of the family was everything that was good and upright and the other branch everything poor and degenerate. Dr. Goddard called the family Kallikak, from the Greek words *kallos* (καλλος), meaning "beauty," and *kakos* (κακος), meaning "bad." There appeared to be a neat "hereditary" explanation for the degeneration of one side of the family. This is how Dr. Goddard described it:

> Both clans had stemmed from the same remote ancestor—Martin Kallikak, a Revolutionary War soldier—but through two different matings. Martin Kallikak himself, it appeared, was of good stock and after the war had married a proper young Quakeress by whom he had seven children— progenitors of all the "good" Kallikaks. However, before his marriage, and while a-soldiering, Martin had dallied briefly with a feeble-minded tavern maid, who, after he went his way, bore an illegitimate son to whom she gave the name of Martin Kallikak, Jr. This individual grew up to be so wicked and odious that he was known as "Old Horror," and sired ten worthless offspring.[9]

According to Dr. Goddard, all the hundreds of bad Kallikaks were descended from "Old Horror," while the good Kallikaks were descended from the Quakeress. But Goddard did not trace all the Kallikaks, so he did not put his theory to the final test. There are other glaring weaknesses. There was no proof that Martin Kallikak was really the father of the tavern maid's son, and even if he was, there is no known genetic theory that could account for all the descendants of one person having a certain character while all their half cousins without exception had the opposite character. The only reason that can be given for Professor Shockley referring to the Kallikaks is either ignorance of the unscientific nature of the story or a willingness to believe in anecdotes that support his case.

To both Eysenck and Shockley the criminal is propelled by forces beyond his own control. It is a convenient rationalization of the failure of our society to prevent crime and removes any suggestion that crime may, at least in part, be the result of social inequalities. But it is dangerous because it removes from individuals the responsibility for their actions. The idea that the criminal is biologically different seems to have strongly developed following the French Revolution, when those in power became particularly worried about holding down the "dangerous classes." The idea recurs whenever society faces periods of social tension. Leon Radzinowicz, the Cambridge criminologist, writes:

> It served the interests and relieved the conscience of those on top to look upon the dangerous classes as an independent category, detached from prevailing social conditions. They were portrayed as a race apart, morally depraved and vicious, living by violating the fundamental law of orderly society, which was that a man should maintain himself by honest, steady work. In France they were commonly described as nomads, barbarians, savages, strangers to the customs of the country.[10]

To understand the causes of crime, we must look not just at the criminal himself but at the society in which he lives. In Chicago, for example, areas that had a high crime rate in 1900 had an equally high crime rate in 1930, although the population of the area had almost completely changed.[11] This is remarkable because one might expect that the new people living in the area would have a higher or lower crime rate depending on who they were. This suggests that perhaps the environment, with its bad housing and rapid population changes, generates a roughly constant amount of crime. The people who lived in these areas had a low social status with few opportunities to obtain good jobs. The quickest way out of such a depressed environment is crime. The community becomes tolerant of crime, and so children learn criminal methods and values at an early age. Many of them enter the criminal subculture and, through drug rackets, gambling rackets, and so on, become part of organized crime. If crime is simply considered to be the inevitable consequence of people having criminal genes, then society is not likely to make the attempt to understand the social causes of crime. Only when these causes are understood can we begin to prevent crime at the roots.

CHAPTER 9

Twins and Crime

Identical twins Ronald and Reginald Kray ruled London's East End with an organized syndicate of criminals until their gang was smashed in 1969. The Kray twins were sentenced to life imprisonment with a recommendation that they should serve thirty years for the cold-blooded murder of rival gangsters George Cornell and Jack (the Hat) McVitie. Their trial at London's Central Criminal Court was the longest murder trial ever to be held there, and the sentences put the twins, with the Great Train Robbers, into an elite class of big-time criminals.

The Kray twins had been partners in crime since childhood. Together they set up in their first business as dealers in secondhand clothes, learned boxing, and did their military service. Together they ran their first club, The Double R, in London's East End and operated protection rackets. They were together when Ronald shot George Cornell at the Blind Beggar public house in Whitechapel for calling him "a fat poof," and when Reginald stabbed Jack the Hat nine times in the face, chest, and throat while Ronald held him from behind.

Were the Kray twins predestined to a life of crime? Was their psychopathic mentality written in their genetic inheritance? Was there some flaw in their mixture of English, Irish, German, and Jewish blood? Identical twins have identical genes: perhaps the evil nature of the Krays was programmed in their genes and they were born to be criminals and to commit almost identical crimes. They would not agree with that theory themselves. They saw their criminal careers as the only outlet for bright boys born in London's East End slums.

Shortly before they were arrested for the last time they told writer Francis Wyndham: "Psychiatrists and that are always arguing about criminal mentality. There's no mystery. If you haven't got an education, and if you want to make something of yourself, what else can you do? There's only boxing other than crime and you can't do that for long." [1]

The relationship of the Kray twins was so intimate and they worked so closely together that it might be said that they were bound to live similar lives. A single case can prove nothing, but a study of many different twin pairs might prove something. It might answer the question of whether criminals are born or made, whether the Krays were born with a killer instinct or were just never taught the difference between right and wrong. Geneticists have attempted to answer these questions by studying the lives of criminal twins such as the Krays.

The first serious attempt to discover if people are really born to a life of crime was made in the late 1920s by Professor Dr. Johannes Lange, who was departmental director of psychiatry at the Kaiser Wilhelm Institute for Psychiatry in Munich. His work still provides the classic evidence for those who believe in a predominantly hereditary theory of the causes of criminality.

Lange's observations were written up in the form of a book—which proved to be popular—called *Crime As Destiny;* the title fairly summarizes his point of view. Lange states unambiguously that crime originates within the criminal. He discovered thirty pairs of twins, of whom at least one of each pair was a criminal. He found the twins with the help of the Bavarian Ministry of Justice and the Institute of Criminal Biology at Straubing Prison. Thirteen pairs of twins were identical and seventeen nonidentical. In ten out of the thirteen pairs of identical twins, both twins had received prison sentences, whereas in only two out of the seventeen nonidentical twin pairs had both twins been sentenced. The criminal careers of the identical twins were extremely similar. Lange reckoned that a pair of nonidentical twins is sentenced no more frequently than are two brothers or two sisters, and so argued that the social influence of a criminal twin is not likely to turn the other twin to crime. Lange concludes that "these facts show quite definitely that under our present social conditions heredity does play a role of paramount importance in making the criminal." [2] He does, however, admit that environment has an effect, and he allows the possibility of social causes of crime in the environment.

Lange describes the criminal destiny of his subjects with a certain unpleasant condescension, but his prejudices become most evident in the final chapter of his book when he begins to generalize his theory and condemn large categories of people for their near-criminal tendencies. What he seems to be saying is that all the types of behavior of which he disapproves are inherited. This presumably helps him to look upon them with tolerant condescension.

> Types closely related to our subjects are to be found without exception in the large group of psychopathic individuals of all kinds. A large majority of them are weak-willed or will-less. Among the symptoms of such people must be classed their ever-ready tendency to fall into crime, though this does not apply to all cases. Putative criminals constitute only one group of the weak-willed. Numbers of others, who suffer from slight or imaginary disabilities, fill our hospitals or wander about our streets. Masses of them are found in professions of recent origin; they are film actors and supers, pavement artists and hawkers, hole-and-corner reporters and "representatives"; even more particularly wives who find everything too much trouble, and prostitutes who take no real pride in their profession.[3]

Lange's personal prejudices are important because there are so many ways in which prejudices can influence a study of this kind, not merely in interpreting the evidence but also in the way in which it is collected. Lange did all the work himself. He decided whether a particular pair of twins was identical or not, and he studied their life histories to decide whether or not they had criminal tendencies. In most cases there seems to be little doubt about the criminal activities of the twins. However, it is not possible to be absolutely certain whether twins are identical or not just on the basis of examination and measurements, even with the assistance of fingerprints and photographs. It is quite possible that some of the identical twins were really not identical, and vice versa. These objections can be overcome by using modern techniques of identification and using more than one investigator. Separate investigators should be used to assess whether the twins are identical or not and whether they are criminal. Another source of error that is extremely important is the means used to find the twins. One or the other twin is more likely to be in prison at any one time if both are criminal than if only one is criminal—so perhaps twice as many pairs will be found in prison when both twins are criminals. In addition, there are other familiar sources of bias such as the more similar treatment of identical twins from birth so that both twins may be exposed to identical influences, such as neglect, which turn them to crime. Hans Eysenck uses Lange's work as the source of evidence to support his own theory of criminality in his book *Crime and Personality* (chapter 3). Eysenck writes of Lange's data that "they do demonstrate, beyond any question, that heredity plays an important, and possibly vital, part in predisposing a given individual to crime"; and "these empirical . . . figures represent under-estimations rather than overestimations of the role of heredity." He goes on: "Since the evidence is so conclusive and reproduced by so many investigators in so many countries, and since it agrees so much with what might be called the common wisdom of the ages, one might expect that common acceptance had been accorded to it, and that any textbook of criminality would give pride of place to these findings." [4] Eysenck's appeal to the "common wisdom of the ages" rings a warning bell. When science has to appeal to the common wisdom of the ages, it is lost. The common wisdom varies from age to age and from one group to another within society.

Lange's work was endorsed almost without reservation by J. B. S. Haldane, one of the most distinguished geneticists of his day. Haldane called *Crime As Destiny* a masterpiece and appears to have seen it as a blow to the doctrine of freewill, which he identifies with Catholicism. He says:

> An analysis of the thirteen cases shows not the faintest evidence of the freedom of the will in the ordinary sense of that word. A man of a certain constitution, put in a certain environment, will be a criminal. Taking the record of any criminal, we could predict the behavior of a monozygotic [identical] twin in the same environment. *Crime is destiny*. The defenders of indeterminism could at most claim that free-will very occasionally tipped the balance over, and thus counted for something in the long run, but not often enough for its effects to appear in a series of a dozen cases taken at random. And a free-will of this kind is clearly of no practical importance. [5]

Haldane goes on to point out that Catholics in England and Wales in 1930 are more than twice as likely to become criminal as members of other religions, and that this is not a very good advertisement for freewill. This little joke is not really very funny. The presumption is that Catholics stem from inferior genetic stock and therefore are more likely than others to be destined for a life of crime. Many Catholics in England and Wales, of course, come from Irish stock and often have the misfortune to live in the poorest parts of cities in the most unfavorable environments. In one great sweep Haldane prejudges and stigmatizes large groups of people by application of the theory of inborn hereditary criminality. Curiously, Haldane was at the time a member of the Communist party of Great Britain and might have been expected to be prejudiced against a hereditary theory of crime. However, in this case his upper-class English background seems to have been stronger than the political views he acquired.

For any valid comparison to be made between identical and nonidentical twins they must be brought up in a comparable way. If the environment acts at all differently on identical and nonidentical twins, then any comparison becomes at least highly dubious. Few researchers now believe that this requirement can be met at all realistically because the very identity of identical twins invites identical treatment within the home, whereas nonidentical twins may be treated on a much more individual basis.

Few investigators have taken the trouble to look at differences in the environment of twins and the way it affects their lives, preferring to think of the environment as a constant that cancels out in all the equations. The most recent study by Karl Christiansen of the University of Copenhagen (1973) shows how the development of criminal tendencies in pairs of identical twins varies with their environment.[6] Christiansen's study of criminal twins is the most comprehensive yet to be published and shows that the assumptions, as well as the methods, of previous studies are totally unsatisfactory and cannot justify the simple conclusion that crime is destiny.

As in most previous studies, Christiansen found that both individuals of a pair of identical twins were more likely to be involved in crime than both twins of a nonidentical pair. If Christiansen had stopped there and made the same assumptions as other investigators and theorists, he might have concluded that there is some genetic predestination to crime. But Christiansen went on to classify the twins according to their place of birth and their final place of residence. He then found that when the two twins lived in rural areas they were likely to have the same fate, whether they were identical or nonidentical twins. In a small society where everybody knows everybody else, there is little freedom for people to pursue their own lives. The shackles of destiny are hardest to throw off where status is most rigidly defined and a person's expectations most widely known. In country districts it is much more difficult for two identical twins who look virtually indistinguishable to establish separate identities and reputations than for two nonidentical twins—and it is difficult enough for them. In the relative anonymity of the city it is much easier for two twins to develop different circles of friends and avoid being inextricably involved in each other's lives. Social predestination is often a fact of life in country districts but can more easily be avoided in cities where greater variety and opportunity exist.

Two important conclusions can be drawn from the work of Christiansen. First of all, as he puts it himself, development of a criminal way of life depends "to a high degree upon the environment of the twins"—a conclusion diametrically opposed to Eysenck's. Second, his analysis shows that in practice it is probably impossible to estimate the strength of any genetic effect pushing these twins toward a life of crime. The environmental influence is so strong that it distorts methods used to try and estimate any genetic influence. The genetic influence, if it exists, is probably too small to be measured.

The criminal with an established record is innocent in law until proved guilty. This principle of justice is challenged by the view that a criminal may be predestined to a life of crime. When the lives and reputations of large groups of people and their image in the eyes of the world are at stake, science should aim to be as impartial as the law. Unfortunately, in scientific matters the same men may, in effect, act as both judge and jury. The same scientists may first collect the data, then interpret it, and finally act as expert advisers. It is easy for science to give spurious authority to popular theories by making plausible assumptions. This is a disservice to society because it simply confounds issues that are already confused.

CHAPTER 10

Dr. Frankenstein and the "Y" Men

"I knew I was preparing for myself a deadly torture; but I was the slave, not the master of an impulse which I detested, yet could not disobey," [1] says the monster after he has murdered Dr. Frankenstein. The monster Dr. Frankenstein created by nineteenth-century spare-part surgery is the classic psychopath unable to control his fits of violent passion. Hollywood horror films have made this monster the prototype criminal madman who is born evil.

Dr. Frankenstein—the obsessive and idealistic scientist—intends to make a perfect human being, but his calculations go wildly wrong, and the result is a hideously misshapen creature with yellow watering eyes. In the original story written by Mary Shelley, wife of the poet, the monster is harmless at first but is so dreadful in appearance that his creator, Dr. Frankenstein, emotionally rejects him. Unwanted and unloved, the monster roams the world terrifying and murdering people. In Mary Shelley's story it is the fear and revulsion the monster's appearance causes in others that drive him to criminal madness.

The best-known version of the Frankenstein story is the Hollywood horror film starring Boris Karloff as the monster. In this film a new twist is introduced into the plot that completely alters the idea of the story. In the film version the monster is by mistake given the brain of a criminal, so it is no longer inhumanity that drives the monster mad but his biological "inheritance." The cause of the monster's criminal tendencies is an inherently bad brain. The film is brilliant, but it turns Mary Shelley's story upside down, making nonsense of the moral that originally lay behind her story.

In 1931, when the film version of *Frankenstein* was made, the idea that criminals had a different brain structure was still popular. This is apparent, for example, in the work of the British doctor Albert Wilson, who spent a lifetime studying the brains of criminals and in 1929 published a book called *The Child of Circumstance*. Wilson believed that criminals came from tainted stock, and he personally dissected the brains of many criminals in his search for the cause of their degeneracy. He describes examining the brain of a "very degraded murderer" who, he says, had "never developed beyond the ape stage":

> Examining with the microscope the brain of a murderer, I found a remarkable contrast to that of a healthy man of 22 years of age, who, sad to relate, was killed in London by a motor bus. The same might be said comparing this degenerate's brain with the well developed brain of a boy of 5 years of age. In the two normals there were layers of cells and fibres in rich profusion, while in the murderer's brain one cell only was developed to ten or fifteen cells in the normal brain; yet his brain was full size and weighed fifty ounces, and his skull was large and not too thick.[2]

Dr. Wilson believed—like many other doctors and scientists in his day—that crime was caused by a combination of misdirected instincts and bad blood. Alcohol and syphilis were the two "secret poisoners of the race," which destroy the germ plasm and degenerate the breed. Underneath an illustration in Wilson's book showing some inmates of an unnamed institution, Wilson writes: "A group of most revolting perverts and weak minded degenerates, kept in a colony. No cure, the only proper treatment is painless extinction. We must stop this type breeding by sterilization." In another place Wilson writes: "Healthy and selective breeding points the only way to salvation. The state should appoint a marriage bureau under the highest medical skill."[3]

The ideas of Wilson, an Anglo-Scot, are close to those lying behind some of the worst excesses of Hitler's Germany. Scientifically Wilson's ideas were unsophisticated by today's standards, but new ideas with similar political and ideological overtones have appeared again in the more sophisticated biology of the 1960s. The myth of the monster lives on in the modern tale of the "Y-factor" criminal.

The mythical monsters of modern crime are the tall, subintelligent inmates of special prison hospitals for the mentally ill who have been found to possess an extra male (Y) chromosome in every cell of their bodies. By an accident of fate, these people develop from a fertilized egg that has one chromosome too many. They have the genetic constitution XYY instead of the normal XY.

The story of the "Y factor criminals," as the London *Daily Express* later called these men, began with a discovery by Dr. M. D. Casey of Sheffield University, England, that 7 out of 942 inmates of Rampton and Moss Side Special Hospitals in England had extra Y chromosomes.[4] Following this discovery, Dr. Patricia Jacobs of the Medical Research Council's Clinical Effects of Radiation Research Unit in Edinburgh made a survey of the inmates of Carstairs State Hospital, a high-security institution in Scotland for mentally disturbed patients with criminal or violent records. Among a total of 315 patients she examined, 9 men were found who had an extra Y chromosome. This was an unexpectedly high proportion, and so Dr. Jacobs suggested that the antisocial behavior of these men "may be causally related to the extra Y chromosome, rather than, for example, to adverse environmental influences in childhood." [5] A survey of the chromosomes of live-born baby boys in Edinburgh had found 1 with extra Y chromosomes out of a total of 1,100.

The Y chromosome is responsible for the development of the male character, with its extra aggressiveness, and the male sexual drive. Geneticists occasionally find fruit flies with extra X or Y chromosomes, and these individuals are called superfemales and supermales, although it is recognized that they are not in fact particularly strong or fertile. Nevertheless, something of the term *supermale* stuck in the imagination and seemed to fit in with the extra height that the Y factor criminals were found to have.

Further study of the nine Y-factor men found at Carstairs was undertaken by two medical geneticists, W. H. Price and P. B. Whatmore, who found that these men came into conflict with the law at an earlier age than eighteen other inmates of Carstairs with whom they were compared. They also found that Y-factor men were much less likely to commit crimes against the person such as murder, assault, and sexual assault and more likely to commit crimes against property. This might suggest that their criminal tendency is not based on any grudge against people. The home environment of the Y-factor men at first seemed to be better than the home environment of the other criminals in Carstairs, but later studies did not bear this out. Only one of the thirty-one brothers and sisters of the nine Y-factor men had any convictions, and this one conviction was for stealing £5 from an employer, whereas thirteen of the sixty-three brothers and sisters of the eighteen men with normal chromosomes had criminal records, with 139 convictions between them. Price and Whatmore conclude:

> There is no reason to believe that these patients would have indulged in crime had it not been for their abnormal personalities. There is no predisposing family environment, and their criminal activities often start at an age before they are seriously influenced by factors outside the home. . . . This leads us to believe that the extra Y chromosome has resulted in a severely disordered personality and that this disorder has led these men into conflict with the law.[6]

The first reaction of many professional biologists was that science had finally been successful in pinpointing a hereditary cause of crime. The discovery followed the success of geneticists in showing that mongolism was caused by an extra small chromosome, and at first sight appeared to be a logical extension of this scientific approach. However, there is a vast difference between mongolism, or Down's syndrome diagnosed by medical science, and criminality, a condition defined by complicated social and legal considerations. The importance of this difference was overlooked.

The press threw aside such little caution as the scientists had expressed and spelled the message out unambiguously. The London *Evening News,* for example, wrote on August 30, 1967, that British medical researchers had discovered "some unfortunate people likely to be destined to a life of crime from the cradle. They are born with the seeds of crime in them and go 'bad' like rotten apples. No longer will it be possible for courts to condemn every prisoner for turning to a life of crime." [7]

The story as it appeared in the *Evening News* was not an exaggeration of what scientists were saying and writing. The British Medical Research Council itself wrote in its annual report to Parliament for the same year:

> From the study of the men at the State Hospital, Carstairs, the XYY male emerges as an unstable and immature individual *without feeling or remorse,* unable to construct adequate personal relationships, showing a marked tendency to abscond from institutions and committing a succession of apparently *motiveless crimes,* mostly against property. If he is mentally subnormal then he is likely to be a high-grade defective; but it seems unlikely that mental subnormality in itself is an adequate explanation of his behavior, for there were some among the XYY males at Carstairs who were not classifiable as mentally subnormal, yet their pattern of behavior did not differ from that of the recognizably subnormal. When all factors are taken into consideration, especially the virtual absence of delinquency in their families and their early age at first conviction, it

seems likely that the extra Y chromosome has a deleterious effect primarily on the behavior of these men, *predisposing them to criminal acts.*[8]
[Author's italics.]

Serious discussion began in the British press about detecting the
source of crime at its roots in the cradle. Nobel Prize-winner Francis
Crick considered the possibility of an "acceptance test" for children
so that abnormal babies might be rejected within two days of birth.
Nicholas Wade asked in *New Society* if it will be "ethically correct to
let XYY babies live." Kennedy McWhirter appealed in the *Daily
Telegraph* for segregation of "genetic deviants" in strictly isolated
communities where they would not interfere with other prisoners. The
medical correspondent of *The Times* advocated routine chromosome
studies for detecting criminals.

A picture began to emerge of babies and criminals being subjected
to tests that would condemn them, not for what they had done or what
they were, but for the chromosomes they possessed. Little mention
was made of the possibility of slaughtering innocent babies or condemning innocent men. The time could be foreseen when a man would
only be innocent until he was found to have an extra Y chromosome.
Fortunately, screening of large numbers of babies for extra Y chromosomes was not then practical, since each chromosome test takes some
four hours of laboratory time and so a screening program would be too
expensive even if it were feasible in other ways. However, it is always
possible that automation might make tests cheaper and that they might
be more widely used.

As a result of all this brouhaha, several criminals, all of whom seem to
have been murderers, used the fact that they possessed an extra Y
chromosome as a defense. In Los Angeles, Raymond S. Tanner appealed against his sentence of fourteen years' imprisonment for assault
with intent to murder after he had raped and beaten a woman in 1967.
Tanner's counsel argued that he was entitled to an insanity verdict
because the extra Y chromosome had "predestined" him to a life
ruled by aggressive and uncontrollable impulses. The motion of appeal
was denied by the United States superior court judge after evidence
was heard from a psychiatrist that Tanner had only an average score
on a personality test measuring hostility. The judge ruled that the evidence was not sufficient to prove any relationship between the XYY
syndrome and human behavior.

In 1969, in another U.S. case, a geneticist testified that Sean

Farley, aged twenty-six, had an extra Y chromosome. Farley was accused of the murder of a forty-nine-year-old divorced woman. Dr. Edward Schutta, a geneticist, said that an extra Y chromosome had been found to be associated with extreme tallness and aggressiveness. However, Dr. Schutta did not agree with a suggestion made by the defense lawyer that the extra Y was necessarily related to antisocial or criminal behavior. He said, "It can contribute, but by itself it would not be a factor."

Erroneous press reports that mass murderer Richard Speck had an extra Y chromosome were also important in establishing a popular link between the extra Y and crime. Speck killed eight nurses in Chicago in 1967. The Illinois Supreme Court upheld his conviction and the death sentence; no evidence that he had an extra Y chromosome was ever produced.

Another question had to be faced by those who believed in a link between Y chromosomes and crime. There are fifteen hundred men with extra Y chromosomes for every million of the population, and there are only some hundreds of these men in prisons and institutions. What has happened to the other seventy-five thousand men with extra Y chromosomes in Britain and over a quarter of a million in the United States? They are almost certainly living normal lives—perhaps with no more problems than their neighbors. Dr. Park S. Gerald, professor of pediatrics at Harvard Medical School, who is making a special study of the Y-factor people, says that a number of men with extra Y's have been investigated and found to be completely normal, and some have been found to have "superior" intelligence.

The possession of an extra Y chromosome seems to be just one factor which in some cases can cause abnormal growth of the body and nervous system. This may cause subnormal intelligence or personality difficulties as a result of brain damage. Y-factor men who have been studied are more likely to have "intention tremors"—a trembling of the limbs—or asymmetrical bodies. These are signs that the nervous system has been damaged during development. This damage may make it difficult for Y-factor men to control their anger. But it is completely misleading to think of an extra Y chromosome as determining antisocial behavior.

Men who have an extra X chromosome (Klinefelter's syndrome XXY) rather than an extra Y have also been found in larger numbers than might be expected in some institutions. Dr. M. D. Casey found twenty-one men with extra X chromosomes in his survey of the Ramp-

ton and Moss Side Special Hospitals—something like ten times the
number found among the newborn. They did not seem to have any
special differences in behavior from the other inmates. Antisocial behavior, larceny, arson, and indecent exposure are common reasons for
men with Klinefelter's syndrome being in these institutions. Unlike Y-
factor men, they do not seem to specialize in crimes against property
but in crimes against the person. Ironically, the men with the extra Y
(male) chromosome, which is supposed to make them aggressive, are
less aggressive toward people than men with an extra X (female) chromosome.[9] The men with the extra X chromosome have physical peculiarities—small testes, scant body hair, possibly developing breasts—
which may make them more resentful of their fellows and more likely
to be picked upon. The Y-factor men, on the other hand, seem to be
gentle giants who choose to attack things rather than people. But it is
misleading to think of these men as simply inheriting extra maleness
or femaleness—what they get in both cases is an extra chromosome
that has harmful effects on body development.

The connection between possession of an extra X chromosome and
crime seems to be no more direct than in the case of an extra Y chromosome. Extra X chromosomes are no more common among criminals or delinquents than in the normal population. However, increased
numbers of men with an extra X chromosome are found in special institutions for subnormals, although these men are usually found to
have relatively high intelligence. The reason given for their being institutionalized is usually that they have a "behavior disorder."

The most recent findings show that the environment appears to be
predominantly responsible for the abnormal or criminal tendencies of
people with extra X or Y chromosomes. Dr. Casey followed up thirty-
three men with extra Y chromosomes, twenty-one with extra X chromosomes, and nine with both an extra X and an extra Y chromosome
who were detained at Rampton and Moss Side Special Hospitals and
compared them and their families with 150 other inmates and their
families. He found no significant differences between the families of
Y-factor or X-factor men and the comparison group. In all three types,
over half the families had been disturbed in some way or there was
some mental disorder or the loss of a parent. Casey points out that if
the extra chromosome was expected to predispose to mental disorder,
then a relatively lower incidence of environmental disturbance would
be expected in the families of men with extra chromosomes. In all the
groups the proportion of patients whose relatives had convictions was
similar. Dr. Casey concluded:

The results of this work serve to show that the presence of an extra chromosome per se plays only a small part in predisposing to delinquency. Confirmation of this observation will require a great deal of prospective work from chromosome surveys of the newborn, but until this has been done it would seem premature to allow the presence of extra X or Y chromosomes to be used in legal proceedings.[10]

The existence of many thousands of noncriminal men with extra Y chromosomes provided a nagging doubt for other scientists. As early as 1968 a few scientists became worried that after all the theory might not be correct. And Dr. W. M. Court Brown, in whose Medical Research Council Unit at the Western General Hospital, Edinburgh, the theory originated, decided to sound a note of caution. He said:

The only conclusion that can be reached at present about a male with an extra Y chromosome is that, by comparison with an XY male, he incurs some increased risk of developing a psychopathic personality. There is, however, no evidence which indicated that an XYY male is inexorably bound to develop antisocial and criminal traits.[11]

But the myth was by then too well established in the minds of both scientists and laymen to be easily put down.

The greatest danger of serious misunderstanding arises when the Y chromosome theory is taken as a proven example of a general principle, and the unwarranted deduction is made that there is a hereditary tendency in all violent crime.

This sort of thinking is evident in a serious article in *The Times* (of London) written in January, 1972, by Mr. E. P. Bellamy, assistant chief constable of Birmingham. He writes:

It is accepted that identical twins develop similar attitudes and outlook, have the same levels of ability and show the same strengths and weaknesses of character. More recent studies have shown this still to be so, even when the twins have been separated in infancy and received very different forms of upbringing and education. It has also been demonstrated that persons with histories of violent behavior quite often have an additional Y chromosome in their blood. There is therefore a degree of scientific support for Mr. Mark's [London's police chief] contention that ''violence is inherent.'' [12]

A scientific study at Harvard Medical School has begun to follow up Y-factor babies to find out what happens to them when they grow up. Dr. Park S. Gerald and Dr. Stanley Walzer, a psychiatrist, say that most Y-factor babies ''are developing into wonderful kids,'' although some ''seem to be impulsive and have difficulty in controlling themselves." [13] However, the ethical basis of this study was challenged by a group of young Boston scientists calling themselves Science for the People. They pointed out that there was a danger that the study could influence the way parents treated their children. Parents might treat their children more "negatively" if they were told the child had inherited an extra Y chromosome. This would harm the child and bias the study. The Boston scientists also criticized the way in which consent was obtained from parents for the project. The dispute was taken up by Harvard's Standing Committee on Medical Research, which ruled that the project was ethical and should be continued.

Dr. Walzer argued that parents had a right to know this research information because it put them in a position to make changes in the child's life and help him in any way possible. On the other hand, it can be argued that there is no positive advantage in knowing that a person has an extra Y chromosome when there is no specific treatment recognized for the condition. Also, it can be said that people have a right not to know. The same problem arises with people who are found in screening tests to be carriers of sickle-cell anemia—or women with testicular feminization syndrome. They are normal, healthy people, but once they know that they have an inherited condition they may find that they are bound to declare the information to their life insurance or health company. The next they may hear is that their premiums have increased simply because to insurance companies they represent an unknown risk. So it may be an advantage not to know if you have an extra Y chromosome.

Already the search for criminal genes has taken on a new twist. The latest suggestion to come from those who are looking for a link between chromosomes and crime is that men with longer Y chromosomes are more likely to turn to crime or to have personality deviation. The length of chromosomes is easily measured with the microscope. Dr. Johannes Nielsen found that 8 percent of the patients attending a forensic psychiatry clinic in Risskov, Denmark, had large Y chromosomes, as compared with 1.4 percent of newborn males. Nielsen argues that there is a connection between the possession of large Y chromosomes and crime because he finds that there are more criminals among the brothers and fathers of criminals with large Y chromosomes than among the brothers and fathers of criminals with small Y chromosomes. Nielsen also says that the chances of these patients committing violent crimes is greater than it is for the patients with short or normal-length Y chromosomes. [14]

However, a group of English doctors have found conflicting results. Although they found an unusually large number of boys (18 out of 387, or 3.9 percent) with large Y chromosomes in a reform school, they found only the expected number of men with large Y chromosomes in Wormwood Scrubs Prison (5 out of 200).[15]

These conflicting findings look like another false lead. There are perfectly normal men in the general population with large Y chromosomes, and there are plenty of criminals with small or normal-length Y chromosomes, so the observation does not look like seriously advancing knowledge of the causes of crime.

Theories of criminality framed in terms of inborn defects have a long history and great popular appeal, perhaps because it is comforting to think of offenders as in some way personally inadequate or as monsters incapable of feeling remorse or responding to punishment. The myth of the born criminal has been perpetuated by the Y chromosome story. The image of the tall man-monster destined to crime because he was born with an extra Y chromosome has become part of modern folklore. Although an accumulation of evidence now shows that there is no basis for the original scientific claims, the myth will not die easily.

To present crime as a biological or medical problem has distracted attention from the search for the real causes of crime within our society. The hereditarian approach tends to assume that the social status quo is normal and that any deviation from it is pathological and *a priori* likely to be inherited. This approach has failed to produce any scientific work that has stood the test of time, and it should now be abandoned.

HEALTH

Love is just as vital to healthy human growth and development as food or heredity. A child may grow slowly because it has inherited genes that will make it small, or because it is deprived of love. In 1915 James H. M. Knox, a Johns Hopkins physician, noted that 90 percent of infants in Baltimore orphanages and foundling homes died within a year of admission despite satisfactory physical care. Children cannot live without love.

In 1948 Elsie M. Widdowson, a nutritionist who was serving with the British forces occupying Germany, studied the growth of children in two municipal orphanages. This is now recognized as a classic study showing the importance of loving care for the healthy growth of children. Each orphanage housed about fifty children between four and fourteen. The children in both orphanages had only official rations to eat.

The matron in charge of orphanage A was a cheerful person who was fond of children, while the matron at orphanage B was a stern disciplinarian, although she had a group of favorites. After six months the cheerful matron left orphanage A and the stern matron took it over, leaving orphanage B. During the first six months with the cheerful matron the children in orphanage A grew much better than the children in orphanage B. But as soon as the stern matron left orphanage B, the children began to gain weight and height. At this time the children in orphanage A happened to be given unlimited bread, extra jam, and orange juice, but under the stern matron they did no better than before, although the favorites, whom the stern matron brought with her, shot up in weight and height with these extras.[1]

These are extreme situations, but they illustrate how children do not just grow up by themselves even when the criterion of healthy growth is strictly physical. The simple conclusion is that man cannot live by bread alone. In our society children who do not get sufficient attention from their mothers also fail to grow.[2] The explanation is that the child who is not cuddled becomes withdrawn and mentally disturbed. This causes the child's pituitary gland next to the brain to alter its output of hormones that regulate feeding and growth.

The emotional and psychological stimulation a family provides for its children is as vital to them as the food they eat. The quality of that stimulation may make a difference of inches to a child's adult height. It may also affect whether children get infectious diseases, whether they take to drugs as teen-agers or take to drink a little later, and it may also decide whether or not a person has a mental breakdown in later life. Hereditarians have minimized these social influences by portraying the human body as a hard machine specified by blueprints fixed at conception. This is as great a disservice to humanity as is the position that hereditarians have taken with respect to intelligence. To understand who people are and why they are like that, we must look at their past environment and their human experiences.

CHAPTER 11

Smoking, Drinking, and Drugs: Innate Depravity?

People who smoke or drink may choose to blame an innate human weakness for driving them to it. If they were supermen, perhaps they would not be such slaves of the habit. Presumably the ideal superman would not smoke, drink alcohol, or take drugs because if he did he would lose absolute control over himself. It is often convenient for the smoker or drinker, who thinks he should give up for health reasons, to believe that his habit is the result of fate.

In 1965 Hans Eysenck brought smokers the message they most wanted to hear. In his book called *Smoking, Health and Personality* he developed the theory that lung cancer is caused by heredity rather than by smoking cigarettes. Cigarette manufacturers were immediately interested in the theory because, if true, it would enable them to shift the dreadful responsibility of causing lung cancer back onto the individual smoker.

Eysenck says that "lung cancer and smoking are related, not because smoking causes lung cancer, but because the same people predisposed genetically to develop lung cancer were also predisposed genetically to take up smoking." Eysenck suggests that smokers are extroverts who have a "stimulus hunger" that leads to a "preference for coffee and alcohol, for spicy foods, for premarital and extramarital intercourse, [for] impulsive and risk taking behavior." [1] Eysenck supported his case with evidence suggesting that smokers were indeed more extroverted than nonsmokers, and that extroversion is a personality trait largely determined by heredity.

Eysenck's speculations, which were well reported in the press, must have given many people the reasons they wanted to carry on smoking. The evidence shows that, in Britain at least, smokers are influenced by such press reports—after each scare there has been a marked drop in consumption of cigarettes and numbers of people smoking. The message came across from Eysenck's book that smoking and cancer are both decided largely by fate. If the theory was correct, it seemed to be of little use to give up smoking, since fate had already decided who would get lung cancer and who would not.

Eysenck's thinking sidesteps some awkward facts. Lung cancer is a modern disease—without cigarettes there would be very little of it. In England and Wales in 1968 lung cancer killed almost 10 percent of men aged over thirty-five, and other diseases caused or aggravated by smoking took a terrible toll. Some thirty thousand people in Britain and seventy thousand in the United States die every year from lung cancer, mostly caused by cigarettes. Many more are disabled by heart disease or bronchitis—sometimes for as long as ten years before death brings relief. Much of this is caused by smoking. If a smoker gives up the habit, however, the chances of recovering or remaining in good health improve steadily, as do the chances of not dying from lung cancer or other diseases caused by smoking.

Eysenck's theory has never been generally accepted by medical experts because of lack of any convincing evidence. His book was published after eight committees of experts in five different countries had concluded that cigarette-smoking is an important cause of lung cancer and other diseases. Few serious scientists now dispute that smoking causes lung cancer and is contributing to heart disease and bronchitis.

And the experience of British doctors who gave up smoking is quite contrary to Eysenck's fatalistic theory. A careful analysis made by Doll and Hill in 1964 shows that the number of deaths from lung cancer among British doctors has decreased progressively as the doctors have smoked less. When the connection between cancer and smoking was first suggested, British doctors gave up smoking in larger numbers than other sections of the population. Doctors were not hard to convince that smoking harms health. Between 1951 and 1965 about half of British doctors who used to smoke gave up, and the number of doctors who die every year from diseases related to smoking has since declined by about eighty. This is an enormous saving in skilled manpower for Britain, in addition to a priceless saving of human life. The study also shows that after a person has given up smoking for ten years, however long he or she has smoked up until then, the chances of dying are little greater than those of someone who has never smoked.[2] Tobacco smoke damages the cells of the lungs—particularly those cells bearing cilia that sweep dirt from the lungs. So smoke particles accumulate in the lungs of smokers, causing the irritation that leads to bronchitis and cancer. When a person gives up smoking it appears that the lungs slowly begin to recover, because the lung cells of ex-smokers have been found to be relatively normal.

Nevertheless, Eysenck does appear to have been right on one point. There is now scientific evidence that some people are very much more likely to get lung cancer than others—*but only if they smoke*. A fortunate 45 percent of people inherit a resistance to lung cancer. But inheritance of the resistant gene appears to have no connection with whether someone becomes a smoker or not. A blood test devised by cancer researchers in the United States is now being used to identify people who carry a gene that makes them susceptible to lung cancer if they are also smokers. The test has been developed by Dr. Charles Shaw and a husband-and-wife team, Dr. Gottfried Kellerman and Dr. Mieke Luyten-Kellerman, working at the University of Texas at Houston. The test is performed by ''growing'' white blood cells for five days in benzpyrene, a constituent of cigarette tar that is known to cause cancer. The test identifies three types of people who conform to the three possible combinations of two genes.

The enzyme detected in the white blood cells of the unfortunate nonresistant people converts benzopyrene, and similar chemical substances called polycyclics, into cancer-causing agents. According to the theory behind the test, white blood cells in the lungs convert polycyclics into agents causing cancer. The theory is highly plausible, although it still remains to be proved.

RR people are resistant to lung cancer. Their white cells do not react to the benzopyrene by forming an enzyme that changes benzopyrene into another substance that is a much more powerful cancer-causing agent. They are the fortunate 45 percent.

PP people are predisposed to lung cancer if they smoke. The tests show that their white cells form increased quantities of the enzyme. Ten percent of people are PP.

RP people have both genes and show an intermediate reaction in the test. They are certainly many times more likely to get lung cancer than RR people, but researchers are not yet sure if they are as highly predisposed as PP people. PP and RP people do not seem to be any more likely to get other types of cancer.

However, the discovery of a genetic predisposition to lung cancer

lends no real support to Eysenck's theory. People who have this predisposition and do not smoke do not get lung cancer, and they are not
in any way predisposed to take up smoking. Indeed, there has never
been any real evidence that anyone is predisposed to become a
smoker. The only respectable study of smoking in twins was made by
James Shields (published in 1962), and this was quite inconclusive
because the sample of twins was highly selective. Many remained in
touch with each other despite separation and so were likely to be similar in their smoking habits. It is always possible that a genetic predisposition to smoking exists, but it has not yet been satisfactorily
proved.[3]

Eysenck returns to the issue of smoking in his book on *Race, Intelligence and Education*. He concedes that he was wrong about the
inheritance of lung cancer, which was the subject of 95 percent of
Smoking, Health and Personality and the mainstay of his theory. Eysenck then changes his interest to heart disease and suggests that
smokers have a hereditary predisposition to heart disease. He is worth
quoting at length:

Many empirical studies have found a strong correlation between smoking
and various diseases, notably cardiovascular and respiratory; official reports from respected bodies like the Royal College of Physicians have
argued that this correlation spells causation, and that the studies quoted
demonstrate that smoking causes these diseases. In "Smoking, Health
and Personality" I pointed out that the evidence was equally compatible
with an hereditary model, and quoted evidence to show that personality
factors, themselves known to be largely hereditary, were associated both
with the development of such diseases as lung cancer, and with cigarette
smoking; it seemed possible that heredity might predispose some people
both to smoking and to diseases. The evidence, therefore, was ambiguous, and could not be interpreted with the confidence shown by the
College of Physicians; what was needed was not more of the same kind
of old-fashioned research which in the nature of things could not bring
forward proper proof of a causal type, but research taking into account
the genetic hypothesis. Such research has now been done, and we know a
good deal more than we did before. Cederlof, Lundman, Friberg, and
their associates have studied tens of thousands of identical twins, one of
whom was a smoker, the other a non-smoker; in these comparisons heredity has been held constant (because in each pair of identical twins
there are no differences in heredity, both having inherited the same set of
genes) so that any differences found would be due to smoking. What was
the outcome? No differences between smokers and non-smokers were
found for cardiovascular diseases (such as coronary heart disease); thus

by eliminating genetic factors, the correlation between smoking and cardiovascular disease was also eliminated! For respiratory diseases the conclusion was quite different; here, differences between smokers and nonsmokers remained, even in the twin sample, proving that this correlation was indeed associated with a direct causal connection.[4]

The research quoted by Eysenck [5] that appears to demonstrate that smoking is not an important cause of heart disease is extremely dubious. It has been criticized by experts in the field, including the United States Department of Health, as well as the Royal College of Physicians of England. Although Cederlof believed that his figures showed a hereditary influence in heart disease, they do not show a consistent trend. Two further studies by Cederlof also fail to provide convincing evidence for the hereditary theory of heart disease, and other studies quoted by Eysenck as supporting the theory are equally equivocal.

Close examination of the evidence shows that there is no basis for Eysenck's original theory. Extroverts may smoke more frequently than other people, but this does nothing to establish any causal relationship between heredity and smoking. Neither is this information of any use in predicting who will become a smoker and who will not. The report of the Royal College of Physicians *Smoking and Health Now* says:

> Cigarette smokers have been found, on average, to be more extroverted than non-smokers. Although the differences are highly significant, statistically they are small, and there is a great overlap between smokers and non-smokers, so that personality characteristics do not reliably predict which individuals will become cigarette smokers. Claims that smokers tend to be more anxious, emotionally tense, and neurotic have not been substantiated.[6]

Is the observation that smokers have a slight average tendency to be extrovert just another piece of useless knowledge? At present it seems to be little more.

Eysenck, who described himself as "fairly introverted," smoked quite heavily at one time. But he was able to give up and is recorded by the London *Sunday Times* color magazine (April 5, 1964) as saying: "There was no psychological therapy, I thought it was highly undignified to be the slave to a habit."

Many people begin to smoke because their friends are doing it and they want to belong to the gang—it is a sign of bravado among schoolchildren, who use it partly as an act of defiance. People continue to smoke once they have started because they are hooked on nicotine, which is mildly habit-forming. When smokers attempt to give up, they

often experience great distress. They are anxious, irritable, and restless, and have disturbed sleep, difficulty in concentrating, and an upset
stomach and bowel, together with an intense craving to smoke. If the
smoker is then given injections of nicotine, this will temporarily relieve the symptoms, but only at the cost of postponing the day when
the smoker is free of his craving.

Something like half of smokers admit privately that they would
like to give up, but there is no simple way of doing it. Tranquillizers
and other drugs such as lobelline do not seem to help much. Some
people say that hypnotism and group therapy help, but this is difficult
to prove. One of the most effective ways of getting people to give up
smoking is for a doctor to advise them that they should do so. Some
30 percent of smokers who have been unable to give up any other way
are able to do so after such professional counseling.

It is extremely difficult for someone to give up smoking when all
his or her friends and family are smoking. It is best, if possible, to
avoid situations where everyone is smoking for the first few days or
even weeks after giving up. Advertising does a great deal to link
smoking with particular social events, times of day, or rituals such as
drinking, so that a smoker finds it difficult to think of having a cup of
coffee or a glass of beer without having a cigarette. Advertising also
links smoking with ideas of manliness, romance, and good living, thus
making young people feel that they are not getting the best from life if
they do not smoke.

The insistence of Eysenck on a hereditary factor in smoking has
distracted attention from the importance of advertising in encouraging
smoking. Although the number of cigarettes smoked has decreased
following press scares—for example, after the publication in Britain of
a report of the Royal College of Physicians on smoking in 1971—the
number always creeps up again after a year or two, showing that advertising slowly neutralizes the effect of press reports of the health
risks of smoking. So long as tobacco companies continue to advertise
their products they must be held responsible for the hundreds of thousands of people who suffer disease and death every year through
smoking.

Alcoholism also provides a battlefield for the heredity-environment
conflict. Very few Jews and Chinese are alcoholics, but alcoholism is
relatively frequent among the Irish. This is a popular observation, but
it is also backed up by statistics. A striking example is the rejection
rate for military recruits in Boston, Massachusetts, during the Second
World War. Three percent of Irish, 1.2 percent of Italians, and 0.2

percent of Jews were rejected for alcoholism. That means alcoholism was fifteen times more common among Irishmen in Boston than among Jewish men. Is this due to the different heredity of these two ethnic groups? It would not surprise a biologist to find that the difference was hereditary. It might perhaps be the result of some inborn difference in the ability of the body to break down or otherwise tolerate alcohol. Indeed, various strains of mice and rats are known that have marked differences in their preferences for alcohol.

However, there are large differences in the way alcohol is used by different societies and social groups, and it is equally possible that the difference in the numbers of Irishmen and Jews who are alcoholics is a result of some difference in culture rather than a result of differing tendencies toward ''innate depravity.'' It is fairly normal for an Italian or Frenchman to drink a large glass of wine with his midday meal, but to many Britons or Americans this would seem peculiar. Similarly, the habit of taking cocktails without food before a meal seems peculiar to the average Italian.

Nevertheless, in all countries the alcoholic is recognizable. The French alcoholic may tend to drink continuously all day without ever getting drunk, and the Anglo-Saxon alcoholic may be more inclined to drink in excessive bouts of drunkenness followed by sober periods. However, the final effect on alcoholics is the same whatever the nationality or race: they drink repetitively in a way that injures their health and interferes with their social and economic functions. Alcoholics all over the world are helpless in the face of alcohol and suffer because of it. Chronic alcoholism is an extremely serious disease affecting about five million people in the United States and perhaps a million in Britain. In France, where a large proportion of the population is employed in industries associated with the production or sale of alcoholic drinks, the proportion of alcoholics in the population is even greater.

Alcoholism does run in families. Various studies have shown that between 10 and 30 percent of the fathers and brothers of alcoholics and 2 to 10 percent of their mothers and sisters are also alcoholics. This percentage is higher than would be expected in the general population. But there is good evidence that the reasons for alcoholism running in families are environmental rather than genetic. In 1945 sociologist Anne Roe studied the fate of children of alcoholic parents who were adopted into other families after intervention by the State Charities Aid Association of New York City.[7] The children she studied were white and were up to ten years old when adopted, which gave them plenty of opportunity to be influenced by the environment of their original alcoholic parents. Anne Roe compared the fates of thirty-six children whose real fathers were classified as heavy drinkers with twenty-five adopted children whose parents were normal.

The alcoholic fathers were overaggressive and disorganized, could not keep a job, and neglected or mistreated their wives and children. A quarter of the fathers were criminal, and three were sex deviants. Only four of the mothers were considered normal, five drank heavily, and half were sex deviants. About half the children had been neglected or mistreated by their mothers. Nevertheless, none of the children adopted into other families showed any signs of alcoholism by the age of thirty-two, although ten of them did have problems of delinquency in late adolescence. Two of the children in the control sample also had problems of delinquency.

The higher frequency of problems in adolescence among the children of alcoholics probably reflects the fact that they were adopted at an older age (an average of five and a half years as opposed to two and a half years in the control children). The home was also important. Anne Roe comments that none of the children taken from their alcoholic fathers and placed in a satisfactory home became alcoholics.

A more recent study of adopted children of alcoholic parents has claimed to find a hereditary factor in alcoholism.[8] However, the results of this study have been severely criticized [9] and the U.S. government report *Alcohol and Health* has urged caution in the interpretation of the findings. The government report said: "Since alcoholism is probably even more than IQ a 'plastic' type of human behavior, the role of heredity in its causation is indeed more difficult to establish . . . the most that can be said safely seems to be that alcoholism may be a familial disease." [10] That is to say the disease may be transmitted in families but not necessarily through the genes.

A child or teen-ager's observation of the way parents use alcohol is probably the crucial factor influencing later drinking patterns. When a child is introduced to alcohol by its use in social rituals in the home, or at meals and celebrations where drinking is restrained and supervised, the child is most likely to become a normal drinker. One highly vulnerable group of people is the youngsters who first begin to drink late in their teens outside the home: they more often become heavy drinkers in later life. Studies of the way Jews use alcohol suggest that their low rate of alcoholism is a result of two factors: their first introduction to alcohol is most often in a sacred religious context, and this is reinforced by being taught respect for alcohol within the family.

As Jews drift away from Orthodox Judaism they are more likely to have problems with alcohol.

Drinking alcohol to excess can be looked upon as a symptom or as a disease. It may, of course, begin as one and lead to the other. Alcoholics may be disturbed in other ways, which may be the primary cause of their drinking. A follow-up study of 250 delinquent boys in Somerville and Cambridge, Massachusetts, showed that 11 percent were alcoholic twenty years later according to a strict definition (hospitalization or member of Alcoholics Anonymous). These boys had been outwardly more self-confident than other children of their age. They had weak family ties and outwardly were particularly independent. Nevertheless, the follow-up showed that in later life they were excessively dependent on their families. The conclusion of this study, made by W. and J. McCord, was that drinking enabled the boys to present a facade of masculinity while remaining highly dependent.[11] The balance of evidence at the moment suggests that alcoholism and psychiatric conditions that may precipitate it are caused by factors in the environment. Predictably, Eysenck is of the opinion that alcoholism "has a marked genetic component."[12]

Since addiction to hard drugs became common in recent years, repeated suggestions have been made that there may be a hereditary factor in drug addiction. In the past, drug addicts have been described as "constitutionally immoral," "hereditarily neuropathic," "nomadic," and "weak in character and will"[13]—all terms implying an *inherited* tendency to take drugs. And some psychiatrists refer to an "addictive personality" as if it were inherited. One suggestion is that there are drug receptor sites in the brain and that addicts may be born with more of these receptors. Such a theory is perfectly tenable, but as yet there seems to be no direct evidence in favor of it. With the continued failure of governments to control the sale and distribution of hard and soft drugs in all countries, the hereditary theory of drug addiction may be expected to grow in popularity. If officials can point to hereditary factors as being responsible for drug addiction it may appear to relieve them of the responsibility to ask why policies of control have failed and whether they should consider some more radical approach to the problem.

However, evidence already exists to suggest that the problem of addiction to hard drugs is a social one and that, given a favorable environment, the majority of people will not become addicted. It used to be an accepted truth about drug addiction, taught in many medical schools in the past, that once people have tried a hard drug they get an insatiable craving for it and are almost instantly and irretrievably hooked. This myth has now been dispelled as a result of the experience of U.S. soldiers in Vietnam.

The heroin epidemic among U.S. soldiers in Vietnam was at its peak in the middle of 1971. Late in that year, troop strengths in Vietnam were rapidly reduced and thousands of soldiers were returned to civilian life. President Nixon made it compulsory for all drug abusers in the army to be given treatment and rehabilitated. There were fears that if these men were returned to civilian life untreated they might become involved in criminal activities in order to obtain heroin supplies. An official survey of the enlisted men leaving Vietnam during the one month of September, 1971, when the drug epidemic was at its peak, was made for the Department of Defense by Dr. Lee Robins, professor of sociology in psychiatry at Washington University, Saint Louis. He found that 20 percent of soldiers leaving Vietnam in September, 1971, said they had been dependent on heroin at some point during their tour of duty, while only 1.3 percent had felt drug-dependent at some point since their return home.[14] This proportion is similar to the 1.2 percent of drug abusers who were identified before military service.

The inescapable conclusion from this study of drug abuse is that in one environment—Vietnam—soldiers will become dependent upon drugs, but this dependence will usually disappear when they return to their familiar environment. For the majority of people at least, there is no inevitable predisposition to abuse these drugs. It is possible, although there is no evidence for it, that the hard core of less easily cured addicts do have some genetic peculiarity making it more difficult for them to give up. On the other hand, it seems more likely that they continue with drug use because they move into an established drug subculture in civilian life.

There do seem to be particular types of personality that are vulnerable to addiction. Many drug addicts seem to have preexisting personality disorders often described as immature, inadequate, or sensitive and passive. In a classic study, psychologist H. E. Hill found, using a standard test, that addicts had socially deviant personalities—that is to say, addicts do not accept the aspirations and goals of the bulk of their fellows. This sort of person is not interested in the ordinary social pursuits and feels little guilt or anxiety if he or she does things that are not socially acceptable. Other studies have shown that the addict tends to have a mood of depressive pessimism, a low self-regard, and a poor ability to maintain relationships with others.[15]

One of the most convincing explanations why people become addicted to drugs has been given by psychiatrist Abraham Wikler of the National Institute of Mental Health, Lexington, Kentucky. He suggests that injection of an opiate drug such as morphine or heroin relieves what he calls "primary needs" such as hunger, fear, pain, and sexual urges. The drug addict obtains gratification because the drug damps down these primary needs. But gradually gratification becomes associated with taking the drug itself and the person becomes physically dependent. Each time the addict experiences withdrawal symptoms, which are satisfied with a shot of the drug, he reinforces this conditioning process.[16]

Since the Second World War there has been an explosion in drug use among underprivileged racial minority groups living in deprived conditions in the United States. Although the large majority of illicit drug users may be negroes, there is also a substantial proportion of whites who take drugs. Poverty, crime, and lack of expectations are among the factors consistently associated with drug addiction. But extreme personal problems and mental disturbance are probably the more common root causes of drug addiction. In Britain the parents of drug addicts are more likely to be divorced, criminal, alcoholic, or mentally disturbed than are the parents of nonaddicts. However, in the United States drug-taking in urban slums has become a way of life for some people, and since it provides employment in an environment that often has little else to offer it may not necessarily attract the same type of person.

A study of heroin use in the slum areas of New York by anthropologist Edward Preble of the New York School of Psychiatry and economist John J. Casey of Georgetown University makes the point that in this environment heroin addiction is "anything but an escape from life." They say that the addict can often be recognized by his fast and active walk because he is always occupied with getting more supplies or evading the law—what the heroin user calls "taking care of business." Preble and Casey question the view of the addict as passive, with an "inadequate personality." They see drug use as a highly organized form of productive behavior, although they agree that it is basically antisocial. They made their study on the Lower East Side and in Harlem, Yorkville, and the Bronx, and they present evidence that the typical heroin user in those areas may avoid violent crime if there is no gain, but if there is the prospect of gain he is probably prepared to use more violence than a nonaddict. Preble and Casey argue that the drug culture is an attempt to make sense out of life, which makes no

sense any other way. They say, ''If the drug user can be said to be addicted, it is not so much to heroin as to the entire career of the heroin
user.'' [17]

The drama of heroin abuse distracts attention from the fact that the
drug that has been most commonly abused in the United States is the
tranquillizer Valium, according to the U.S. government survey Project
Dawn. In Britain, Valium is probably too easily available to be abused
in the legal sense but there is no doubt that it is being overprescribed
and often for people who are better off without it. For example, Dr.
Christopher Ounsted wrote to the *British Medical Journal* saying that
nine out of ten women who came to his battered-baby clinic in Oxford
were on tranquillizers such as Valium, or antidepressants prescribed
by their doctors. The first step he took in rehabilitating these mothers
and their babies was to take them off these drugs and substitute old-
fashioned nursing care and understanding advice. Tranquillizers have
an effect on the brain similar to that of alcohol—they can make a person feel more relaxed when he is in the right mood, but if a person is
tense they may make him violent. So a mother who is given tranquillizers without any extra support or change in circumstances is more
likely to batter her baby. What might really do the mother some good
would be to enable her to get away from her baby more often in the
evening and go out for a social evening with her husband.

It has taken society thousands of years to learn how to use alcohol,
and we still abuse it badly. The ancient Hebrews are recorded as having a problem with drunkenness around 500 B.C. but now there are
fewer alcoholics among Jews than any other group of people in the
West. They have absorbed the use of alcohol into their culture and
regulated its use within the family for social and religious occasions.
This example shows how drugs can be regulated by social conditioning and social pressures. It is extremely difficult for governments to
encourage this sort of use of alcohol in the face of entirely uncon-
trolled advertising. If use of drugs and alcohol is to be regulated
socially, then advertising must be carefully controlled and parents
must be told the best way of introducing their children to alcohol.
There is evidence that people who drink moderately benefit in the
sense that they live longer than total abstainers. This may not necessarily be because alcohol has any direct effect in prolonging life, but
rather because abstainers are more often tense, unrelaxed people who
therefore suffer more nervous strain. An official U.S. government
report on *Alcohol and Health* pointed this out and recommended a

"safe level" of drinking of not more than one and a half ounces of alcohol a day—that is, about half a bottle of wine, two pints of strong beer, or three and a half whiskeys—which should always be well diluted.[18] This quantity was first recommended by a Scotsman, Dr. Francis Anstie, in 1864 and is still known as "Anstie's limit." [19]

My own prescription for reducing abuse of alcohol and tobacco would be to ban all advertising of them. Some people will see this suggestion as a threat to the rights of free enterprise, but I see it as leaving the individual free from commercial pressures to make up his own mind about whether he wants to drink or smoke. This would make it much easier for a social consensus to emerge, which I hope would exercise some restraining control over patterns of drinking and smoking behavior. To control use of medically prescribed drugs, the public needs to understand much more about their real effects. The medical profession has only recently become aware, for example, of the way in which sleeping pills change normal brain activity during sleep and the way tranquillizers can make people aggressive. When these messages get across, the demand from the public for these drugs may eventually decrease. The problem of heroin and hard drugs is a special one, and here we need much more research by sociologists to discover how life in our cities may be changed so that the drug culture is less attractive to young people. It is doubtful if much more can be done than contain the hard-drug problem without making radical improvements in the quality of life for people living in our inner-city areas.

CHAPTER 12

The Predisposition Theory of Disease

Man is a savage animal—this was the belief of many social thinkers in the nineteenth century who were influenced by Darwin's theory of evolution. Only the fittest would survive. Those who were weak or diseased came from degenerate stock and would be eliminated by nature. Some eugenicists were not satisfied with the rate at which natural selection weeded out the weak and were intent on speeding it up.

In Germany, Ernst Haeckel, professor of zoology at the University of Jena, deplored the role of doctors who kept alive patients with tuberculosis, syphilis, and mental disease. Haeckel called for the present generation of the diseased to be eliminated so that future generations would be free of these diseases.[1] In England, Karl Pearson, one of the founding fathers of British genetics, lumped people with tuberculosis together with other "undersirables," and in 1911 he wrote: "Every segregation which reduces their chances of parentage is worthy of consideration."[2] Pearson believed that "the diathesis of tuberculosis is certainly inherited, and the intensity of inheritance is sensibly the same as that of any normal physical character yet investigated by man."[3] This belief was common in the nineteenth century, though it had been badly shaken by the discoveries of Pasteur and Koch. There could no longer be any doubt that tuberculosis was caused by the tubercle bacillus, but there was still difficulty in explaining why some people got the disease and others did not. This can now be satisfactorily explained by knowledge of the processes by which people become immune to the disease, but the importance of immunity was not properly understood by Pearson and Haeckel.

The view that tuberculosis was the result of hereditary weakness was most convenient to those who wanted to do nothing to improve the lot of the poor who lived in slums. Hereditarians such as Pearson repeatedly emphasized the existence of a hereditary element in tuberculosis and advised that any environmental changes would be useless. This can only have delayed important public health measures that later were to greatly reduce the incidence of tuberculosis long before the miracle drugs became available.

Now that tuberculosis can be cured there is not the same fear of it, nor the shame that people and their families used to feel when they knew they had a disease supposed to be caused by bad heredity, nor is there much interest in the question of whether it is hereditary or not. Nevertheless, the idea that tuberculosis is hereditary has persisted—despite a lack of convincing evidence—and can be found in recent textbooks of medical genetics. It would not surprise doctors or biologists today if susceptibility to tuberculosis were inherited, since hereditary susceptibility to disease is well known in experimental animals. However, a review of the scientific literature shows that there has never been any really good evidence to show that a hereditary predisposition to tuberculosis does exist in man.

A hundred years ago in the crowded cities of Europe, tuberculosis killed hundreds of thousands of people a year—more than any other disease. It was picturesquely called "the captain of the armies of death" and "the great white plague." In Britain around 1898, tuberculosis killed seventy thousand people a year, but by 1948, half a century later, less than twenty-seven thousand people a year died from TB, and today the figure has been reduced to a few thousand.

Today several drugs are available to treat tuberculosis and vaccinations can give immunity to the disease. But improvements in the environment have been at least as important in reducing the incidence of the disease. Certification of dairy herds to prevent the sale of milk contaminated with the bacteria causing tuberculosis, campaigns against spitting in public places, the mass X ray and general improvements in living conditions in cities have all helped to reduce greatly the incidence of the disease.

Before Koch discovered in 1882 the bacterium that caused tuberculosis, the cause of the disease was obscure. It was thought to be due to contagion, but as it was commonly observed to run in families a hereditary factor was also suspected.

Tuberculosis was commonest among the lower classes, particularly in the city slums, and people were ashamed to admit having the disease because it was so often associated with poverty. Perhaps to compensate for this and to account for the frequent cases of young people in better families dying of the disease, the idea arose that tuberculosis was a sign of genius, which made the premature deaths of young people much more poignant. So many eminent poets, writers, philosophers, musicians, and artists died of the disease that the idea was not difficult to support. Dostoevski, Goethe, Voltaire, Samuel Johnson, Molière, Schiller, and Chekhov are a few of the brilliant men who have suffered from it. It is also possible that the experience of the disease itself may have helped to stimulate the imaginations of these artists, through long hours in bed too exhausted to do anything but fantasize. And perhaps long hours of inactivity during periods of remission and convalescence allowed the tuberculosis patient to develop his powers to a peak of genius not obtained by others. However, tuberculosis was so common in the past that its occurrence in so many distinguished people is probably no more than coincidence.

The idea that there is a hereditary influence in tuberculosis has persisted to this day, although the idea that it may be associated with genius has been dropped. As with diseases such as cancer and mental illness, which are also looked upon with fear and shame, there may be a certain comfort for the healthy in believing that "bad heredity" is at least partly responsible for the suffering caused by the disease. The superficial similarity between mental illness and tuberculosis and the shame attached to tuberculosis have been pointed out by Dr. Emil Rothstein of Tufts College of Medicine in Massachusetts as recently as 1956:

> The diseases are both insidious in onset and, although one is caused by a specific agent, the basic reason for a patient's falling ill in either case was and is rather obscure. Mild cases might be expected to recover, severe ones rarely. Neither disease is viewed objectively by the lay public; each is considered as somewhat shameful, for which excuses and apologies must be made. Heredity is popularly considered an important cause, as well as other more mystical factors.[4]

As with the early studies of twins and crime, the early studies of twins who suffered from tuberculosis appeared to show a strong inherited susceptibility to the disease. However, these studies were made by Nazi sympathizer Professor Otto von Verschuer and others in Germany in the period just before the Second World War, and the twins were collected from hospitals and sanatoria in such a haphazard way that a proper scientific analysis cannot be made.

The first survey of any importance was made in 1943 by German émigré geneticist Franz Kallman in New York. He collected twins in a more systematic way, although the sample was far from being representative. He concluded after analysis of some 78 identical and 230 fraternal twins that "the chance of developing tuberculosis increases in strict proportion to the degree of blood relationship to a tuberculosis index case." [5] He calculated that the chances of an identical twin getting the disease if the other twin had it were at least 3.5 times greater than it was for fraternal twins. Similar results showing a less dramatic effect of heredity were obtained in 1956 by B. Harvald and M. Hauge in Denmark. [6]

These studies are still quoted in textbooks as evidence for a hereditary factor in tuberculosis. However, a later study made in 1963 by Dr. Barbara Simonds for the Prophet Committee of the Royal College of Physicians showed that the existing data on twins and tuberculosis could be interpreted quite differently. On the face of it, her study was evidence for a hereditary factor in tuberculosis. However, she went on to test the hypothesis that the greater chances of suffering from tuberculosis among identical twins were the result of a greater similarity of their environments. [7]

If there were such a thing as hereditary predisposition to tuberculosis, then identical twins would be expected to develop tuberculosis whether they were in the same house or not. Dr. Simonds compared the incidence of tuberculosis in identical twins living apart from their tubercular twins and found no significant difference in the numbers who had contracted tuberculosis. She also observed that the chances of a husband or wife of a twin getting tuberculosis were no different from the chances of a blood relative (twin, parent, brother, sister) getting it.

She concluded that there was no evidence for a hereditary factor in tuberculosis and that an identical twin was simply more likely to be exposed to infection if his or her twin became infected.

There is another recent example of the hereditary theory of disease being preferred to the environmental theory. In 1970 it was suggested that some people have a genetic susceptibility to the virus that causes hepatitis B (a type of jaundice). This theory, like the susceptibility theory of tuberculosis, has not been substantiated by the facts. Hepatitis is commonest among poor people, blacks, and people from tropical climates. It is now being recognized that hepatitis spreads among these people because of their unsatisfactory living conditions, and that when these conditions are improved, they are no longer so susceptible.

If cures could be found for the other human conditions associated with hereditary taint—crime, insanity, and low intelligence—then interest in hereditary aspects of these conditions might greatly decrease too. However, since the environmental causes of crime, mental illness, and low intelligence are much more complicated than the causes of tuberculosis, it is not such a simple matter for governments to legislate to diminish them, as governments have succeeded in doing with some infectious diseases.

Many rare diseases really are caused by heredity. They are rare because the people who have these diseases do not have many children and often do not survive until the age when they might reproduce. Hemophilia is one of the best-known examples, and phenylketonuria, a mental defect caused by an abnormality of body chemistry, is another. Others are hereditary deafness and dwarfism. Genetics has made an enormous contribution to the understanding of these diseases, particularly, for example, mongoloid idiocy, or Down's syndrome, as many doctors prefer to call it now. An important piece of scientific history is attached to this change of name. In the past, mongoloid idiocy was explained by a racist evolutionary theory: mongols were said to be "throwbacks" to a more primitive stage in the evolution of our race.

Mongols have a low intelligence level and small slanting eyes with an inner skin fold that gives them a superficial resemblance to people of the Mongoloid race. In fact, mongols are found in all races, including the Mongoloid and Negroid races. Mongoloid idiocy was first described by Dr. John Langdon Down, a physician at the London Hospital, in 1866.[8] He distinguished the various types of idiocy and suggested a classification on racial grounds. Some idiots he considered were of the Ethiopian (negro) type, others of the Malay type, others akin to the American Indian, and so on. This theory remained popular until at least the 1930s and was not finally discredited until 1959, when French scientist Dr. Jérôme Lejeune discovered that mongols have an extra chromosome in every cell of their bodies. This extra chromosome is the cause of their abnormal development. Mongols get their extra chromosome by an accident of heredity, caused simply by two chromosomes sticking together during the formation of the egg cell. This accident of heredity is commoner in babies who are born to older mothers, although the reason why is not exactly known.

Allergies are caused by the interaction of a person's inherited constitution with some factor in the environment such as pollen or chemical dust, although psychological factors such as an emotional upset may sometimes trigger an attack. This is why some people suffer from hay fever or allergic asthma and others do not. There may be many similar variations in the immunity system that provides the body's main defences against disease.

Inherited deficiencies in the ability of the body to produce antibodies in the blood or white cells to fight invading bacteria and viruses are now well known, and people who suffer from such deficiencies are generally susceptible to a wide variety of diseases. It seems likely that deficiencies that make a person susceptible to certain particular diseases such as tuberculosis, leprosy, or certain types of cancer may also exist—but these inherited predispositions will be quite different from the type of general susceptibility to tuberculosis that has been postulated previously. They will probably be comparatively rare conditions associated with rare and atypical types of disease.

Many inherited diseases only appear under certain environmental conditions and cannot be so easily explained as hemophilia or mongolism. Often the exact nature of the hereditary defect is not known, nor are the factors in the environment that precipitate the disease. Huntington's chorea is an example of a hereditary disease that may strike at any time between the ages of twenty and fifty or even later in life, causing gradual destruction of cells in the brain, with uncontrollable fits and often madness. A person steadily deteriorates after the onset of the disease and dies. At present there is no known cure. Woody Guthrie, the folk singer, died of it after thirteen years of degenerating illness, his last years spent paralyzed in an institution, unable to speak or feed himself. The moving story of this desperate illness is told in the film *Alice's Restaurant,* and his son Arlo still does not know if he or his two children will inherit the disease.

There are few good examples of inherited resistance to disease unique to a particular race. Most instances where such differences have been suggested in the past have almost always been accounted for by differences in immunity. Diseases such as polio, tuberculosis, or measles are usually relatively mild if caught in childhood. But if one of these diseases is caught by an adult who has never been exposed to it the result will be much more severe. When measles was first introduced into the Sandwich Islands, for example, many thousands of people died. There may be racial differences in susceptibility to measles between Europeans and Pacific Islanders, but this has certainly never been proved. Occasionally white settlers have taken advantage of such lack of immunity and used disease deliberately as a sort of biological warfare: an example of this is white settlers deliberately selling blankets infected with smallpox to American Indians.

Settlers have an interest in presenting native people as basically weak and unable to withstand the hardships of "civilized" life.

The most outstanding example of racial differences in susceptibility to disease is the sickle-cell gene carried by about 10 percent of American negroes and up to 20 percent of some African tribesmen. This gene has been found to be commonest in the areas of Africa where malaria is prevalent, and it appears to give the person who carries it some resistance to malaria. The direct cause of malaria is, of course, a parasite carried by mosquitoes.

When two people with the sickle-cell gene have children, on average one quarter of the children will inherit two copies of the gene and thus have sickle-cell disease. This is a severely disabling anemia, and people who have it usually die young before having children. The sickle-cell gene confers an advantage on those who carry one copy of it by making them resistant to malaria, which prevents the gene from being reduced to a low level in the population by means of natural selection. However, in the United States, where malaria has been virtually eliminated, the gene is no longer an advantage to those who carry it, and so the gene may be expected to die out slowly, over a period of many years.

People often fear that cancer is inherited, but there is no evidence that this is so for the vast majority of cancers. Cancer is such a common disease that it is quite common for several people in a family to die of it simply by coincidence. Dr. Francis Roe, a cancer research expert at the British Tobacco Research Council, calculates that there is a one in twelve chance that four or more members of a family of eight will develop cancer of one type or another sometime in their lives. Some rare forms of cancer are inherited. One of these affects the eye and causes about 1 percent of cancer deaths in children. This disease, called retinoblastoma, can be cured if it is detected early, and fortunately the disease usually only affects one eye. A person who has retinoblastoma is likely to pass it on to half his or her children.

Cancer has many causes. Viruses may be a contributory cause, but there is little evidence that cancer is spread by infection in the ordinary way. Viruses suspected of playing a part in causing cancer are relatively common and cause a person to develop cancer only when something else goes wrong too. For example, a chemical present in food or mineral oil constantly irritating the skin might, in combination with a virus infection, cause a cancer to begin. But for the cancer to grow, the body's resistance must be low, at least temporarily. Cancer experts now believe that new cancer cells frequently appear in the body but the body weeds these out by means of its normal defenses, which destroy "foreign" cells in the same way that they destroy infecting bacteria. The body's immune defenses may be low when a person is subject to stress and strain, and so it is not incredible to suggest that stress may be an important factor in causing cancer.

The high incidence of stomach cancer among the Japanese might be thought to have a hereditary racial basis if other information was not available. Stomach cancer is commoner among Japanese living in the United States than among whites. However, Japanese living in Hawaii suffer more stomach cancer than Japanese living in the United States, and Japanese living in Japan have the highest rates of all. This all points to an environmental cause—presumably a difference in diet. It is only comparatively recently, however, that much attention has been paid to such evidence. Previously, different incidences of disease among different races have commonly been put down to racial and hereditary factors.

Similar observations suggest that there may be important environmental causes of such common conditions of Western populations as heart disease, bowel cancer, diabetes, stomach ulcers, and appendicitis, which, together with lung cancer, are among our commonest diseases. More people are dying of these diseases than ever before. It is often assumed that this is simply because people are living longer now that so much infectious disease has been conquered, but this explanation is too simple. This is undoubtedly a factor, but it might just as reasonably be asked why, proportionately, more people do not live to die of genuine old age. Medical researchers are beginning to look at all aspects of Western diet, from sugar and refined carbohydrates to dairy produce and animal fats, in search of causes of these diseases, which cut people down before they reach their full life-span.

Some rare cancers of the colon are known to be hereditary. But the majority of the cancers of the bowel are not. Dr. Dennis Burkitt, Medical Research Council fellow in London, has studied the relationship between bowel cancer and diet and has observed that bowel cancer, diverticular disease, and appendicitis are common in communities with a refined diet.[9] These diseases are rare in communities with a diet containing a lot of fiber. Fiber is the celluloselike roughage present in fruit and vegetables and particularly in "brown" cereals (brown rice, whole wheat, etc.). The diet of most Western countries contains very little fiber. White bread, for example, contains almost none: the bran or brown husk of the wheat is removed before white flour is milled.

Diseases believed to be caused by a highly refined diet have been called the "diseases of civilization" because they are so rare among people in rural communities living on unprocessed food. The commonest type of diabetes may also be largely a result of eating excessive amounts of sugar. There may be a genetic factor in diabetes too, but this is probably of comparatively little importance in the type of diabetes that starts in middle life. The frequency of diabetes in Western countries has been steadily increasing with increasing consumption of sugar, although it declined temporarily as a result of food shortages during the Second World War. The importance of this trend has not yet been fully appreciated because it probably takes something like twenty years for someone on a high-sugar diet to become diabetic. This is also the approximate length of time it may take a smoker to get lung cancer.

There is a parallel between these dietary diseases of civilization and smoking, which, in its own way, is also a disease of civilization. We have a reluctance to question the virtue of habits that are an established part of our life-style. And these bad habits are also defended by the special interests of major industries with highly effective publicity machines: the tobacco and alcoholic drink manufacturers, the flour millers and bakers, the sugar producers. The serious consequences of tobacco smoking are now accepted by all, but the debate about sugar and dietary fiber is still in the early stages. Conclusive proof that diets containing large quantities of sugar and refined carbohydrates cause these diseases of civilization is still wanting, but the evidence collected so far arouses grave suspicions. Before the final proof is obtained, a great deal more argument about the genetic nature of these diseases may be expected. If genetic cause could be established, it would shift responsibility for these diseases away from society and the manufacturers onto the individual sufferers.

CHAPTER 13

The Causes of Mental Illness

In 1788 King George III became seriously ill. He was confused, talked to himself incessantly, and had hallucinations. There was widespread speculation that he had gone mad. Physicians puzzled over whether the king suffered from "original madness," which was thought to have a poor expectation of cure, or from "consequential madness," which might be expected to subside with a change in the underlying cause. Several of the king's doctors believed that his madness would prove to be temporary, but after the condition lasted for some months, doubts increased. The king then recovered and reigned for another ten years without a serious attack, until in 1801 he was stricken again and remained ill for the last ten years of his reign. Many believed that George III was insane and that the House of Hanover was tainted with hereditary madness.

American psychiatrists in the nineteenth and twentieth centuries confidently pronounced that King George III suffered from manic-depression, and this diagnosis was largely accepted by historians until it was questioned a few years ago by British psychiatrists Dr. Ida Macalpine and Dr. Richard Hunter. After an exhaustive examination of original sources they came to the conclusion that George III suffered from a physical illness called porphyria.[1] As a result, historians have had totally to reassess the character of the king, and in a small but important way history has had to be rewritten. As long as the king was thought to be insane, his every action was given the worst interpretation and whatever he did was thought to be done for the wrong reason.

The diagnosis of porphyria—a physical disease that causes delirium rather than insanity—enables the historian to be more sympathetic in evaluating the king's influence on political affairs. The symptoms of porphyria are caused by the presence of large quantities of chemicals called porphyrins circulating in the blood. As a result of an inborn error of body chemistry in people with the disease, porphyrins are made in their liver and bone marrow in unusually large quantities. These porphyrins circulate in the blood to the brain and derange its normal function, so that even today people suffering from porphyria are often thought by doctors to be suffering from mental illness. In one large series of cases of porphyria, 12 percent were legally certified as insane. However, the disease can be recognized in many cases because the skin becomes sensitive to sunlight and porphyrins are secreted in the urine, giving it a bluish color. It was these characteristic symptoms which enabled Dr. Ida Macalpine and Dr. Richard Hunter to trace the disease back in the royal line to Mary, Queen of Scots, and down in the other direction to two living descendants of the Hanoverian line who were found to have increased quantities of porphyrins in their urine.

Porphyria is extremely rare or nonexistent in most parts of the world, but about 1 percent of the Afrikaner people of South Africa suffer from the disease. All these people appear to be descended from one Dutch settler who went to Cape Town in 1686 and, like many of his descendants, raised a large family. Porphyria is inherited in an irregular way. The symptoms of the illness are not the same in every person who inherits the gene. Some people may show no symptoms at all but pass the gene on to their children, so that the disease skips a generation or two. Environmental factors are also important in affecting the severity of porphyria. The course of the disease is quite often mild until the sufferer takes barbiturate sedatives, which make the condition very much worse. Unknown factors in the diet may also bring on an attack. Dr. John Brooke, a historian, describes how King George III has been maligned:

> His firmness during the American war in adhering to a policy which was unwise and ultimately disastrous, but was undoubtedly supported by Parliament and public opinion, was considered as the result of an inability to face reality—a defect in his personality which ultimately drove him insane. His moral qualities during these years, which in more fortunate circumstances might have been virtues, were degraded into vices. His perseverance in supporting what he (and the majority of the nation) believed to be the right of Parliament was pathological obstinacy; his courage, a re-

fusal to face facts; his loyalty to his ministers, a wish to govern by corruption. So long as it was believed that he suffered from insanity every aspect of his life and character was seen in a distorting mirror. Even his fidelity to his marriage vow was turned against him, and he was reproached for sexual timidity, presumably because he did not have mistresses. No doubt had he been as loose in his morals as his father and grandfather this would also have been taken as pointing to mental instability.[2]

In assessing the influence of mental illness on a man's life, the values of the historian appear to reflect those of everyday life. As soon as someone is pronounced mad he must often face a devaluation of himself. If someone who at first apppears to be mad can be shown to be suffering from a physical illness he suddenly obtains our sympathy. A person suffering from physical illness or temporary madness still commands some sympathy, but a person with hereditary madness commands only pity: such a diagnosis appears to carry so little hope. This is why the search for the causes of mental illness has become such an emotionally loaded issue. And it has been impossible for researchers to separate the question of what causes mental illness from the entirely different question of who is to be blamed for it: the patient, his parents and friends, or society as a whole.

There are a few other rare hereditary conditions causing mental derangement or madness. Children born with the disease phenylketonuria become mentally deficient—often with IQs under twenty—because of the excessive production of phenylpyruvic acid in their bodies, which interferes with the growth of the brain and the nervous system. If these children are spotted early enough and given a diet containing only small quantities of the damaging phenylpyruvic acid, they can be saved. However, once the damage to the nervous system has occurred it is not possible to reverse it. In the United States and Britain it is now routine for newborn babies to be tested for phenylpyruvic acid in urine or blood before they leave the hospital. And if the test is positive, then they are put on a diet right away.

Only the gene that causes a predisposition to a disease is inherited, not the disease itself. The disease itself may never occur if the environment does not also favor it. Nevertheless, diseases such as phenylketonuria or porphyria are inherited and under average conditions will follow a predictable course. The existence of such diseases caused by defects in body chemistry—the so-called inborn errors of metabolism—has inspired scientists to look for similar causes of schizophrenia and other mental illnesses.

Schizophrenia is a common disease, affecting something like 2 percent of all people at one time or another. Most people know somebody who has suffered from it, although they may only have been told that the person was suffering from nerves or mental breakdown. When Eugen Bleuler, one of the founding fathers of psychiatry, coined the word *schizophrenia* in 1908, he described it as "a specific type of alteration of thinking, feeling and relation to the external world." [3] Such alterations in thinking and feeling characteristic of schizophrenia pose great problems for doctors and scientists who have studied the disease, because of the great difficulty of being certain that a diagnosis is correct.

Many psychiatrists prefer to think of schizophrenia as a pattern of symptoms rather than as a single disease. When a person is schizophrenic, it is often difficult to establish an emotional relationship with him. Literally, the term *schizophrenia* means "split mind." This does not mean dual personality but a separation of the schizophrenic person's thoughts from the reality of his or her own body and surroundings. A schizophrenic man will often refer to himself as "he" rather than "I." To another person a schizophrenic talks a mixture of jumbled-up sense and nonsense mixed with strange fantasies and absurd patterns of words. Schizophrenics may have delusions of grandeur or of persecution (paranoid schizophrenia). The schizophrenic person may be highly intelligent but quite unable to apply his or her intelligence while going through a period of insanity.

A healthy and attractive girl who has always been a fair worker starts to get into trouble at her job for slackness and inefficiency. She starts to take days off for no apparent reason and sits at home doing nothing. Over a period of months she shuts herself off from her friends. She refuses to get up in the morning and spends all day in her nightgown. She neglects to wash herself or comb her hair and sometimes stays in her room all day. When anyone is able to get near enough to talk to her she reveals strange ideas. She believes that her thoughts are no longer her own but are being put into her head by others. She spends hours waiting for personal messages that she believes will be broadcast to her over the radio, but when a message comes it is ambiguous and she does not know what she has to do. When she is by herself she has vivid thoughts that she hears so clearly that they sound like voices. She believes that someone is trying to suffocate her with poison gas or perhaps by a death ray focused through the television set. Eventually her behavior is so disturbed that relatives call the doctor and she finds herself in a mental hospital. She is suffering from a "schizophrenic breakdown."

The symptoms of mental illness vary from one culture to another, and also within one culture over a period of time. A person who is mentally ill is looking for a credible metaphor through which to express feelings and experiences. Religion used to provide this metaphor, but with a decline in the observance of religion there has been a decline in religious mania, although it may be increasing again now, because of the rise of new religious cults. The discovery of X rays and radio waves has been accompanied by a rise in manias expressed in pseudoscientific terms, such as space travel, unseen flying objects, or hallucinations of receiving messages on cosmic rays. For some reason, it has become less common for patients to be seen standing frozen like statues. Beneath all these differing symptoms lie the same basic mental disturbances.

To approach the search for causes of mental illness scientifically, it is first necessary to be reasonably certain that there is some agreement about who is mentally ill, or schizophrenic, and who is not. It is only in very recent years that psychiatrists have found a way of formulating this most fundamental question.

When psychiatrists talk about the major categories of mental illness such as schizophrenic and depressive illness, are they talking about the same thing? A team of British psychiatrists investigating why there were so many schizophrenic patients in mental hospitals in New York compared to London discovered that psychiatrists in the two cities were making their diagnoses on entirely different criteria. The term *schizophrenia* was being used so readily in New York that it was almost a substitute for the words *mental illness*.

However, when an international team approach to diagnosis was used, the number of patients diagnosed as schizophrenic in the New York hospitals dropped dramatically and the number of schizophrenic patients in the London hospitals also dropped, but only slightly. Apart from schizophrenia, the only other illnesses diagnosed at all commonly in the New York hospitals were depression (7 percent) and alcoholism (12 percent). In London only one third of patients—half as many as in New York—were classified as schizophrenic and many more than in New York (one third) were classified as depressive.[4]

The team of British psychiatrists was able to explain the large numbers of schizophrenics in New York only after an elaborate check

on methods of diagnosis. Interviews with eight selected patients were
recorded on videotape and shown to psychiatrists in London and New
York for diagnosis. There was broad agreement between psychiatrists
on both sides of the Atlantic over three of the cases, which were more
or less typical schizophrenia, but about a quarter of the British psychiatrists chose to call three less typical cases of schizophrenia "affective
psychosis." There was serious disagreement over the last two patients:
the majority of the Americans diagnosed schizophrenia, whereas the
British psychiatrists diagnosed either personality disorder or neurotic
illness. One of these patients, a woman, was diagnosed as schizophrenic by 69 percent of American psychiatrists but by only 2 percent
of British psychiatrists.

This study of psychiatric diagnosis has now been extended by the
World Health Organization to include seven other countries.[5] The
United States and Soviet Russia were found to be seriously out of step
with all the other countries in their diagnoses: they classified patients
as schizophrenic who would be considered to have only a minor mental illness or to be sane in other countries.

The findings of the survey substantiate the increasingly frequent
accusations that psychiatry in both the U.S.A. and the USSR is being
abused. American psychiatrists such as Thomas Szasz, professor at the
State University of New York and author of *The Manufacture of Madness,*[6] point out that three times as many people are committed to
mental hospitals in the United States as in the USSR. Hitherto Szasz's
views have been considered by many psychiatrists to be rather extreme, but since the WHO report, published in 1974, they will have to
be taken more seriously.

The WHO report shows that in the United States "symptoms"
such as homosexual preoccupation, passivity, and social inadequacy
are given much higher priority in the diagnosis of mental illness. Psychiatrists in the United States use different rules of diagnosis from the
rest of the world and include in the term *schizophrenia* ordinary neurosis, personality disorder, and mania. Obviously the rules used for
diagnosis are to some extent arbitrary so long as the experts who have
regular dealings with each other understand what is meant. The criteria
used in the United States can be criticized, as Szasz has done, for
labeling people as crazy when they are simply neurotic. They can also
be criticized for exaggerating the importance of homosexuality in diagnosis of mental illness, since many homosexuals are well-adjusted
people.

The wide variation in the diagnosis of mental illness, and the changes that have taken place over the years within the United States, call into question much of the research done into the inheritance of schizophrenia and other mental illness up until 1973. We cannot be sure that the various groups of psychiatrists researching the inheritance of schizophrenia have been talking about the same thing, and we must question how objectively they defined the term for themselves.

Researchers who have come to psychiatry from other sciences have not been in a good position to puzzle over the problems of diagnosis. The biochemist wants to be told which person is schizophrenic and which person is not, and then he will say whether he can find a chemical difference between them. This hard approach of the so-called exact sciences often pays dividends—the naïveté of a researcher moving from one field to another can sometimes pay off. The biochemists cannot be blamed for not knowing that the term *schizophrenia* had such a soft definition. Research into the biochemistry of this disease has a long history of failure relieved only by what seems to be never-ending optimism.

When molecular biology was beginning to become influential in the 1950s, the idea became popular that mental illness was probably the result of a defect in molecules in cells of the brain. The slogan "no twisted thought without a twisted molecule" was coined. The slogan was a play on words, referring to the twisted strands of the DNA molecule—the genetic material—and to the "twisted" protein molecules produced by a defective gene. The idea gained credence because of theories suggesting that a single gene might be the cause of schizophrenia and because of observations suggesting that drugs such as amphetamines and LSD can induce hallucinations and temporary madness. The suggestion was that schizophrenia was caused by an accumulation of some substance similar to LSD in the blood and brain, so causing hallucinations and the muddling of thought. This postulated substance—like porphyrins or phenylpyruvic acid—accumulated in the body and was secreted into the urine because the schizophrenic person was supposed to have inherited a defective gene. The defective gene produced a defective enzyme molecule (biological catalyst), which could not get rid of the postulated substance fast enough by the normal process of breaking it down into some other molecule.

These theories were presented at scientific meetings and in scientific literature with missionary zeal. It looked for a time as if chemistry would discover the cause of schizophrenia in one big breakthrough. However, as hard data began to pile up they were found to be inconclusive. No one ever seemed able to clinch any of the biochemical theories.

Riding on the crest of this wave of enthusiasm for twisted molecules, Sir Julian Huxley and other geneticists suggested in an article in *Nature* that schizophrenia was a "genetic morphism." They wrote: "Tests are beginning to provide evidence of a detectable 'mauve' and 'pink' factor in the urine of a large majority of schizophrenics." [7] The pink substance referred to was DMPEA, a chemical related to LSD and mescaline, that may cause hallucinations. The novelist Aldous Huxley, brother of Sir Julian, had described the intensified and distorted view of the world obtained under mescaline in his book *The Open Door*. This possibly influenced his brother, Julian, and may have given him the original idea for the theory.

Over the next few years biochemists and doctors increasingly found what they were looking for in the urine of schizophrenic people. Pink, purple, mauve, red, yellow, and even gray spots were found. The only embarrassment was the increasing number of claims. In 1966 one scientist recorded the intellectual intoxication of the time: "There was a remarkable consensus that the molecular basis of schizophrenia was firmly established. The specific details of the biochemical pathology still must be spelled out, but no scientist prepared to listen to evidence can continue to insist that schizophrenia is not a molecular disease." [8]

Ten years later science is still waiting for the "specific details" to be spelled out. The "spot" theory of schizophrenia is now no nearer to being established scientifically than it was in 1966. The biochemical approach ran into difficulties when it became clear that people in mental hospitals had different constituents in their urine because they were living on different diets or because they were taking drugs. The substances in a person's urine vary with the bacteria in the bowel and the frequency with which the bowel is emptied. A constipated person might, for example, have a different set of spots in his urine from a person whose bowels are regular. Furthermore, the various spots at first thought to be peculiar to schizophrenics have all been found in the urine of a proportion of normal people. The "spot" theory has never lacked advocates, but the evidence so far has been unconvincing. One distinguished geneticist, Professor J. H. Edwards of Birmingham, England, remarked: "The pink spot now appears to be a red herring." [9] Other biochemical theories of schizophrenia have suffered an equally ignominious fate. Many modern theories about the inheritance of schizophrenia originate from the old theories of the eugenic school of psychiatry. Hans Luxenburger, Bruno Schulz, Franz Kallman, Erick Essen-Møller, Erik Strömgren, and Eliot Slater—some of the most distinguished researchers in human genetics and psychiatry—all studied under Professor Ernst Rüdin in Munich before the Second World War. Several of them were forced to flee from Nazi Germany, while Rüdin busied himself with other experts advising Heinrich Himmler how to draft laws for the sterilization of the unfit and the exclusion of Jews from the state. However, the approach of Rüdin's students to the study of heredity in psychiatry has been more rigorous and scientific. They have patiently refined the crude methods used by the old eugenicists. But despite the devoted work of this generation of men we are little nearer to having any certain evidence that schizophrenia is inherited biologically.

In several early studies of identical twins, it appeared that if one twin had schizophrenia, then the other one would also develop the condition in 70 percent of cases. However, this type of result was obtained only for schizophrenic twins discovered through hospital lists. When the twins are obtained from surveys of the general population they are much less likely to share the same history of mental illness. As in studies of inheritance of criminality, the evidence obtained for inheritance of schizophrenia has declined in strength as observations have steadily become more carefully controlled.

Schizophrenia does run in families, however the term is defined. If a person is schizophrenic there is a greatly increased chance—8 or 9 percent—that a brother or sister will also be schizophrenic. If one parent and one child are schizophrenic there is a 12 percent chance that another brother or sister will be schizophrenic, and if both parents and one child are schizophrenic then the chances are 35 percent. These facts are not in dispute. The question is what causes this increased chance of schizophrenia in certain families.

The strongest evidence for the hereditary theory of schizophrenia is often said to come from studies of identical twins who have been reared apart. If the cause of schizophrenia is hereditary, then despite separation into different environments both identical twins would be expected to become schizophrenic—at least in the majority of cases. However, identical twins who have been reared apart are rare. Only seventeen pairs of identical twins, one or both of whom are schizophrenic and who were separated near birth, are known in the world.

Those who support the hereditary theory of schizophrenia tend to lump all the seventeen separated "schizophrenic" twins together and then claim that as a whole the evidence supports the hereditary theory.

But this is unjustifiable because of the different ways in which the twins have been found, and simply leads to absurdities. A higher proportion of all the seventeen separated twin pairs are both schizophrenic (eleven pairs) than in several series of identical twin pairs who have not been separated. But twins who are not separated would be expected to be more similar, as has been found in studies of other characteristics. The evidence from identical twins separated in early life—which is often quoted as among the most important evidence in favor of a genetic cause of schizophrenia—is too scanty and unsystematic to be reliable. And it is doubtful if large enough numbers of separated "schizophrenic" twins could ever be collected in an unselected way to give a statistically valid result. The only possible conclusion at present is that it is perfectly possible for one separated identical twin to be normal and the other schizophrenic, suggesting that some environmental factor is at work.

There are several other ways of trying to identify a hereditary cause of schizophrenia. One of these is to study adopted children who later become schizophrenic. If the cause of schizophrenia is hereditary, then the biological relatives of schizophrenic adopted children would be expected to be schizophrenic more often than the adopted relatives. Such investigations mark a great improvement in methodological approach to the problem and the results are interesting, but once more they have proved inconclusive.

Dr. Seymour Kety, Dr. David Rosenthal, Dr. Paul Wender, and Dr. Fini Schulsinger, working at the National Institute of Mental Health, Bethesda, Maryland, and the Psychological Institute at Kommunehospitalet in Copenhagen, found 33 schizophrenics out of 5,483 people who were adopted in Copenhagen between 1924 and 1947. They compared the incidence of schizophrenia in the biological relatives of these adopted schizophrenics with the incidence of schizophrenia in the relatives of normal adopted people with similar backgrounds.[10] It is only by including borderline cases that any kind of argument could be made from the data for the inheritance of schizophrenia. Twenty-three out of 33 schizophrenics who were adopted were chronic or acute cases. But there were no more cases of chronic or acute schizophrenia among their biological relatives than among their adopted relatives.

There is no direct evidence to support any particular genetic theory of schizophrenia, although there are several genetic theories consistent with the facts. Theories suggesting that a recessive gene is the cause of schizophrenia can be ruled out because the incidence of schizophrenia is much the same in parents as it is in brothers and sisters of schizophrenics. If schizophrenia were caused by a recessive gene, then the incidence among brothers and sisters would be very much higher than in parents. This leaves the genetic theorists with two possibilities: schizophrenia may be caused by a dominant gene or it may be caused by several genes acting together.

If schizophrenia is caused by a dominant gene, a special subsidiary explanation must be made to account for the fact that the gene sometimes appears to skip a generation. Normally a characteristic caused by a dominant gene carried by one parent will appear in half the children, on average.

If one of a pair of identical twins shows a characteristic caused by a dominant gene, then the other twin would normally also be expected to show the characteristic. However, dominant genes—such as the gene causing porphyria—are known to skip a generation or do not have effects in both members of a pair of identical twins. These genes are called by geneticists "incompletely penetrant."

A gene may be incompletely penetrant because one or more other genes are modifying its activity, or because different environments alter its activity. Invoking such a gene is another way of saying either that the environment is important or that more than one gene is involved in the characteristic—or perhaps both. One of the several genes sometimes postulated to predispose a person to schizophrenia may, however, be more important than others. And it is theories of this type that have obtained most favor because they give some hope that the biochemist may yet be able to identify some particular chemical defect in schizophrenics.

The concept of an incompletely penetrant gene—used in the absence of convincing biochemical data—makes it possible to explain almost any awkward characteristic in human genetics, and there is often no means by which the theory can be readily tested. When a characteristic in an animal is said to be incompletely penetrant it is possible for this to be verified by breeding experiments, but this is obviously not possible with people. Similar objections can be made to theories postulating that schizophrenia is caused by many genes, all of which are equally important: these are called multifactorial or polygenic theories.

Another great weakness of genetic theories of schizophrenia is that they do not adequately explain the large numbers of schizophrenic people in the general population. About 1 or 2 percent of all people in

Western countries are known to suffer from at least one episode of schizophrenia at some time in their life. People who suffer from schizophrenia are less likely to marry than other people, and if they do marry, are less likely to have children. At most, schizophrenic people have on average only 70 percent of the number of children that other people have. Other genetic conditions such as porphyria or phenylketonuria, which are sometimes compared with schizophrenia, are rare. At most one in every ten thousand babies born suffers from one or other of these conditions. The reason they are so rare is that people with these diseases are less likely to reproduce themselves, and so their genes are constantly being eliminated from the population.

There can only be two genetic explanations why a postulated gene for schizophrenia could be so common when the condition itself confers such a disadvantage. The first explanation is that the postulated gene for schizophrenia mutates much more frequently than is normal. This is a possibility with some precedent in the genetics of fruit flies but no known parallel in man. If the postulated gene for schizophrenia did mutate at the very high frequency necessary to account for the facts, it would be unique in human genetics.

The second explanation at first seems more plausible. This suggests that the brothers and sisters of schizophrenics have large families and are also extraordinarily creative people who give their children special advantages that make them more likely to succeed in life and have large families. If this were the case, then the families of schizophrenics might in the end leave as many offspring as the families of other people—so passing on the postulated gene for schizophrenia to future generations. But what evidence there is just does not support this theory—if anything, the relatives of schizophrenics have fewer children than normal.

The hereditary theory of schizophrenia has one virtue: simplicity. It can be readily understood by anyone. Its weakness is the shortage of entirely convincing evidence in its favor, as contrasted with the unambiguous evidence in favor of environmental influences. On the other hand, the weakness of environmental theories of schizophrenia lies in the difficulty of precisely identifying the environmental factors contributing to the condition.

When there is such a wide area of doubt in defining who is mentally ill and who is sane, the one criterion everybody can accept is whether or not a person has spent any time in a mental hospital. However, this is a misleading guide both to the sanity of the people who have never been in a mental hospital and to the relative insanity of those who have been. Immediate actions of relatives and others, as well as more distant childhood causes of mental illness, may contrive to place a person in a mental hospital. And the psychiatrist may often not be certain whether the most insane member of a family is the one who has been committed.

A family or social group decides together whom it will tolerate and whom it will not, under the influence of current ideas about what behavior is acceptable. Those who are not tolerated because of their peculiarities—which may include their political opinions—sometimes end up in a mental hospital. This is particularly evident in Soviet Russia, where political dissidents have drawn the attention of the world to the way they have been imprisoned in mental hospitals.

Cases similar to the Russian dissidents are difficult to find in the West, but they do exist. Ezra Pound, the American poet, was detained in a mental hospital, labeled as incurably insane, for many years after he had made pro-Fascist broadcasts from Italy during the Second World War. Thomas Szasz believes that others such as Marilyn Monroe, James Forrestal, Ernest Hemingway, and Earl Long should also be listed among the people who have been destroyed by a society which did not understand them and stigmatized them as emotionally. disturbed.

If the major cause of schizophrenia is environmental—and there is no scientific evidence yet to compel another view—then society may more easily sympathize with schizophrenics and recognize their problems as its own. But if schizophrenia is found to be caused by heredity, or if this is simply accepted as the current wisdom, then schizophrenics will continue to be given treatment based on the idea that they are fundamentally different from the rest of us. The hereditarian view of schizophrenia, as of other human conditions, looks to segregation and special treatment, whereas the environmental view looks to integration and change of social conditions. Hereditary theories of mental illness are divisive: they separate the sheep from the goats and so create two categories of people. One is considered human and the other is often in danger of being regarded as subhuman.

Genetic causes of mental illness must obviously be recognized if and when they are proven, and special treatment may then be found based on a new understanding of the illness. It is still quite possible that a special category of hereditary schizophrenia will be recognized as distinct from environmental schizophrenia, although at present there is no convincing scientific evidence to suggest this.

CHAPTER 14

Madness and the Family:
Are We Driving Each Other Crazy?

Since the beginning of this century there have been twice as many people in mental hospitals in the Irish Republic as in England and Wales, proportionate to the population. Does this mean that all the sanest Irishmen have emigrated? No, because "madness" travels with the Irish. In New York in 1930 a higher proportion of second-generation Irish were admitted to mental hospitals with a diagnosis of schizophrenia than any other immigrant group. Do Irish people, perhaps, have a genetic predisposition to become schizophrenic? Or is there some peculiarity of Irish culture that increases the chances of Irishmen going insane?

The Protestant Northern Irish have no corresponding increased tendency to become schizophrenic, although they are of mixed Irish, Scots, and Anglo-Saxon stock. Dr. H. B. M. Murphy, a psychiatrist at McGill University, Montreal, found that among fourteen rural communities in Canada schizophrenia was least prevalent among Irish Protestants, whereas it was more prevalent among Irish Catholics than any other group, except Russians and Poles.[1]

The high frequency of schizophrenia among the Irish Catholics in Canada cannot be explained away as a result of the stress of immigration itself, since the Irish at home also have a greater than normal tendency to become schizophrenic. A genetic predisposition to schizophrenia also seems unlikely: the Irish tend to develop schizophrenia before the normal age of marriage, which is late in Ireland. The chances of people marrying and having children are lower once they have had a period of mental illness, so the chances of their genes being passed on to the next generation are also lower. Therefore a genetic predisposition could not account for the high frequency of schizophrenics in Ireland.

Taking this in isolation, it is only possible to speculate on the cause of the tendency for Irish Catholics to become schizophrenic. Catholicism itself may be an important cause. Dr. Murphy has examined the frequency of schizophrenia among other immigrant minorities in Canada and finds that Catholicism is the one common factor associated with increased frequencies of schizophrenia.

Among eight different immigrant minorities studied by Dr. Murphy, schizophrenia was always more common in Catholic than in Protestant males, and in five out of eight immigrant minorities it was commoner among Catholic females than among Protestant females.[2] These figures were taken from official statistics for seven provinces of Canada and derived from the whole population of the provinces, regardless of how many generations the minorities had been in the country. The predominance of schizophrenia among Catholic males of all national origins from Russian and Dutch to Eskimo and French obviously cannot be explained on a racial basis.

Dr. Murphy suggests that Catholic cultural teaching may be at odds with the wider cultural beliefs and demands of society. Protestantism stresses work, independence, and private problem-solving and tacitly approves material aims. Catholicism stresses the community, obedience, and a greater attention to less tangible ideals that may conflict with aspects of contemporary culture.

Dr. Murphy has been able to take the analysis a little further in a study of six Catholic French-Canadian communities. He found an extremely high incidence of schizophrenia among women in three strongly traditional communities, although the communities were in different counties and there had been almost no recent intermarriage. In these very traditional communities the women most often became schizophrenic after the age of thirty-five when their first child is about to leave home, or before marriage when they are trying to establish a career for themselves outside the home. Schizophrenia is extremely rare among young married women, although it is common among such women in less traditional communities.

In the traditional communities, motherhood is an extremely rewarding role and the possibility of a career for a woman outside the religious orders is only slowly being accepted. The ideal woman gets married early and is hardworking and submissive to her husband. But in the last generation the girls have been better educated than the boys. More education has recently become available, but the boys continue to work in the fields while the girls are left to study longer. A conflict appears to have arisen in the minds of many women between their ideals of womanhood and their other goals and expectations of life. The conflict emerges first as an attempt to escape from marriage into a career, or later as an attempt to sabotage the marriage. During the early years of marriage, when the woman is able to apply her education to the bringing up of her young children, the stress appears to be more tolerable.

Similar conflicts may be a cause of schizophrenia in other communities. Dr. Murphy suggests:

In the Polish and Irish Catholic cases from this survey one can detect a clustering of pathology in sections of the communities that are particularly affected by some cultural inconsistency or conflict of expectations, and a relative absence of schizophrenia in other sections of the population whom the culture either demands very little from or guides very clearly.[3]

Murphy implies that schizophrenia is a likely outcome when conflicts affect a person for long periods, so that there is continuing pressure from the community to make a choice together with conflicting advice about what that choice should be. This conflict can affect men more than women in some cultures. In one Polish community in Canada surveyed by Dr. Murphy, more men than women suffered from schizophrenia. In the men it came on early and was severe, whereas in women it came on late and was milder. Apparently Polish tradition expects young men to leave their homesteads and prove their capabilities before being recognized as responsible and ready for marriage. In order to do this in Canada, the young men had to adjust to a modern Canadian way of life, so that while fulfilling the demands of tradition they at the same time lost much of the traditional basis of their lives. So it was difficult or impossible to fulfill the demands of both loyalty and tradition.

The shock of adjustment to a new culture also appears to be the cause of the high frequency of mental illness found in refugees after the Second World War. A group of refugees was taken to Britain from camps for displaced persons in Germany, but despite careful medical screening a remarkably high proportion of them became schizophrenic. Schizophrenia was at least three times more common among these refugees than among British people, and their average length of stay in hospital was longer. In Germany itself the numbers of people in mental hospitals at this time were fewer than in Britain. Increased mental illness in immigrants is often explained as being due to selective migration of susceptible people. However, this explanation does not explain the facts of this case, since the refugees were selected on health grounds and little personal choice was involved in becoming a refugee or in moving to Britain. Any selection on the basis of interviews would have had the effect of excluding schizophrenic people from the group. In some way, the change from refugee camps to resettlement in Britain seems to have caused conflicts and stress that precipitated schizophrenia.

A similar study of U.S. army soldiers, made by Dr. Harry R. Steinberg of Howard Medical School in Washington, D.C., and Jack Durrell of the Psychiatric Institute of Washington, shows that joining the army—whether a person is drafted or volunteers—is a highly stressful experience.[4] More soldiers break down and are hospitalized with schizophrenia in the first few months of service. Battle itself is also a cause of severe psychological stress, as shown by studies of Royal Air Force flying crews during the Second World War. The numbers of psychiatric breakdowns in battle seem to be more closely associated with the degree of danger, as judged by casualty rates, than with the number of missions flown or the degree of physical exhaustion.

The suggestion that stress is a cause of schizophrenia is not in conflict with the genetic theory, since most genetic theories suggest that there must be some factor in the environment, such as stress, that precipitates schizophrenia. Individuals certainly vary in their ability to cope with stress, and in their susceptibility to schizophrenia, but this variation may simply be the result of varying experience of life. There is no reason to assume that the variation is genetic, and the evidence considered in the last chapter certainly does not encourage such an assumption.

But what are the special stresses that trigger schizophrenia? Refugees crowded in camps remain quite sane and able to cope with the most physically trying conditions, but when they are suddenly placed in a strange culture they break down. The stresses that cause schizophrenia seem to be more personal ones, issues that affect an individual most acutely, issues demanding responses for which there is no clear precedent to follow. The complexities of normal life in a totally strange country may impose much greater strains than the circumscribed life and physical hardships of a refugee camp. Stresses are far more intense and more likely to cause mental breakdown when there is no escape from them and they are unrelieved for long periods. When a woman, such as those in the traditional French-Canadian communities, is faced with a continuing conflict between her sex role and her concept of herself, then the strain may only finally be resolvable in mental breakdown. A breakdown postpones what may appear to be an impossible decision.

Other stresses arise from conflicts within the family. The family is in a sense just a special social situation. The theories of schizophrenia that pinpoint conflicts within the family as a cause of schizophrenia all have certain features in common. Confused or even deliberately ambiguous communication that lasts for long periods and affects emotional relationships is often suggested as a cause of schizophrenia. One family member may be most frequently put in this confused and ambiguous position and be unable to escape from the family—or, if he (or she) does escape, may take his confused behavioral responses with him so that he perhaps breaks down much later in life when other stresses have built up.

Over the last ten years a body of evidence has accumulated that points to peculiarities in the family background of schizophrenics that must be at least partly responsible for causing the condition. Gregory Bateson, the distinguished British anthropologist who worked for many years in the United States, suggested in 1956 that schizophrenic people are often caught in what he calls a "double bind": [5] they are constantly put in a situation within their family where they are given confusing and contradictory signals so that, whatever they do, they cannot win. These confusing signals may arise from an ambivalent attitude of the parents to their son or daughter and may be quite unconscious. The ambivalence and confusion of signals are often seen in a contradiction between verbal and nonverbal communication that leaves the person not knowing what to do and finding himself in the wrong if he does anything. The theory suggests that exposure to this treatment over many years leaves a person totally confused so that even the most ordinary exchange may seem ambiguous, and the only escape is into an inner world of fantasy.

Bateson, who worked at the V.A. Hospital in Palo Alto, California, for ten years, gives this example of an exchange between a schizophrenic patient and his mother to illustrate the double-bind situation:

A young man who had fairly well recovered from an acute schizophrenic episode was visited in the hospital by his mother. He was glad to see her and impulsively put his arm around her shoulders, whereupon she stiffened. He withdrew his arm and she asked, "Don't you love me any more?" He then blushed, and she said, "Dear, you must not be so easily embarrassed and afraid of your feelings." The patient was able to stay with her only a few minutes more and following her departure he assaulted an orderly.[6]

If the young man had been able to say to his mother that it was obvious that she had difficulty in accepting a gesture of affection from him, the whole incident might have been resolved—at least for him. But the schizophrenic, according to Bateson, does not have this option open to him because of his intense dependence on his family and training in the family not to discuss such issues explicitly. If the schizophrenic attempts to discuss such an issue, he just ends up being further humiliated. In this particular case Bateson says, "The impossible dilemma [double-bind] thus becomes: 'If I am to keep my tie with my mother, I must not show her that I love her, but if I do not show her that I love her, then I will lose her.' " [7] As a single incident an ordinary person would perhaps find this situation only upsetting, but when the situation is repeated constantly, madness is a not surprising outcome.

Theodore Lidz, professor of psychiatry at Yale University, has pointed to another way in which parents may cause their children to become schizophrenic. The personality of one of the parents may be so fragile that this parent must subjugate the whole family to function in such a way that his or her own precarious integration is maintained. The conception such a parent has of himself or herself does not respond to new circumstances. Reality is excluded in order to maintain the delicate emotional equilibrium. Lidz says:

> The parents' delimitation of the environment and their insistence on altering the family members' perceptions and meanings, creates a strange family milieu filled with inconsistencies, contradictory meanings, and denial of what should be obvious. Facts are constantly altered to suit emotionally determined needs. The children in such families subjugate their own needs to the parents' defenses, and their conceptualization of experiences is in the service of solving parental problems rather than in mastering events and feelings.[8]

Studies made by Dr. Lyman Wynne and Dr. M. T. Singer at the National Institutes of Health in Washington, D.C., have shown that the parents of schizophrenic patients communicate in a peculiar way whether or not the schizophrenic patient is present. One study of 280 families has shown that it is possible for a psychiatrist using special tests and interviews to identify the parents of schizophrenic patients correctly in 90 percent of cases.[9] The experiments were carefully controlled so that it was not possible for the psychiatrist to discover which

parents had schizophrenic children. Neither were these parents themselves schizophrenic.

Dr. Wynne found that parents of schizophrenics have peculiarities
of speech and language usage that are not the same as those of schizophrenics themselves:

> It has been our overall impression that the parents of schizophrenics who
> are not themselves overtly or symptomatically schizophrenic, speak in
> communication patterns which are maximally befuddling to a listener
> who is trying to share a focus of attention with these parents. Tentatively
> our data suggest that the parents of schizophrenics show these features in
> a considerably more pervasive and frequent fashion than the same fea-
> tures are found in the communication of the schizophrenics themselves.
> Schizophrenics show other kinds of disorders, ordinarily features which
> are more easily identified as crazy and therefore can be dismissed or not
> "heard". However, the parents of schizophrenics tend to communicate in
> such a way that the listener tries to understand, but ends up distrusting his
> own understanding.[10]

These theories suggest, in effect, that parents drive their children
mad. Simple as this suggestion has been to some, it has understandably aroused tremendous opposition from parents who are made
to feel guilty for their children's madness. But this overlooks the fact
that the parents themselves are no more responsible for their own personalities than are the children for theirs, and so should not be blamed.

Methods of upbringing and reactions to situations going back over
many generations may culminate by "throwing up" a schizophrenic
person in a particular family. The reason why one person in a family
becomes schizophrenic and not another may sometimes be that that
person is physically weaker. He (or she) may then be picked on as the
weakling. Or a person may be born at a time when the family is going
through a particularly stressful period and so may be picked on as the
family's "whipping boy." However, it is not until the incipient schizophrenic tries to break away from the family in adolescence and establish a life of his own that he experiences his breakdown. For a child
within the family, the crazy relationships somehow work, but they are
useless as a model for learning how relationships function in the world
outside.

"Childhood schizophrenia" or autism is an entirely different condition that has no direct connection with adult schizophrenia. The autistic child is cut off from the rest of the world and appears to want no
contact with anyone, however loving the approach may be. The autistic child can hear but does not listen and can see but will not look di-

rectly at a person. The only emotions he shows are outbursts of rage. The original cause of the condition may be some kind of brain damage at birth complicated by emotional reactions of the family, but this is not certain. It has also been suggested that the cause may be failure of the mother—for example, through illness—to establish a relationship with the child shortly after birth. Whatever the cause, some autistic children now make a good recovery with expert help.

A great advance in the understanding of the problems of schizophrenic people came with R. D. Laing's recognition that crazy people may be talking a kind of sense, if only the listener can find the key to it all. The key often lies in the muddled, and sometimes deceitful, relationships between family members. R. D. Laing and Aaron Esterson showed how such warped relationships can be penetrated in their book *Sanity, Madness and the Family*.[11] They used the method of interviewing the schizophrenic person and each of the near family members, including aunts and uncles when relevant, and they often found that the story that came out in the individual interviews was quite different from the story that came out when the family members were all together. The whole family was often found to be mad in the sense that their relationships had moved away from reality.

In their book Laing and Esterson tell the story of the Edens. Ruby Eden was admitted to a hospital in a trancelike state, behaving as if she were a wax dummy. This is a catatonic stupor, a severe form of schizophrenia. One moment she said she was the Virgin Mary and the next that she was the wife of the pop singer Cliff Richards. She complained of bangings in the head and of voices calling her a "slut" and a "prostitute." She said at one moment that her mother loved her and at the next that she was trying to poison her. She had totally lost her sense of reality. Laing and Esterson ask whether Ruby had really lost her sense of reality or if it had been torn to shreds by others.

After twenty interviews with members of the family in various combinations it transpired that Ruby was illegitimate but that there had been an elaborate conspiracy to keep this knowledge from her. Through no fault of her own she was confused about her family relationships and about who she was. She had been taught to call her uncle Daddy, her real father Uncle, her aunt Mother, and her real mother Mummy. The family disagreed violently over whether Ruby had grown up knowing who she was. Her real mother (Mummy) and her aunt (Mother) said that no one knew the real state of affairs, but her cousin (whom she called brother) maintained that Ruby had known for a long time.

Ruby was surrounded by mystifications. She knew that people (voices) were talking about her, and her family knew that people were talking about her, but they told her not to be silly and not to imagine things. They told Laing and Esterson that she was a "slut" and no better than a "prostitute," but denied such feelings to Ruby and made her feel bad or mad for perceiving their real feelings beneath. The crisis came when Ruby became pregnant and Mummy and Mother got her on the divan and pumped soapy water into her uterus to procure an abortion. They then told her she was a disgrace and that history was repeating itself—so acknowledging her illegitimacy explicitly for the first time. Her uncle angrily told her to get out of the house, and twice she did so, although he denied to her (but not to Laing and Esterson) that he had ever asked her to go. Surrounded by such confusing accusations and denials, Ruby understandably could make no sense of her world. She did not know for certain who she was and she did not know for certain whether the things she heard and perceived were really said or came to her from within (voices). In the end she did the only thing she could, which was to withdraw totally into a catatonic stupor.

Ruby's situation was ultimately unbearable and so she broke down. Other cases of schizophrenia may involve much less easily identifiable sources of confusion than hers. The only criterion that anyone can have as to whether or not a situation is unbearable is a purely subjective one. Could anyone, given a childhood like Ruby, have broken away and worked out a sane life of her own? Do you think that *you,* perhaps with a more stable childhood, have inherited such a tough constitution that you can withstand any amount of emotional turmoil and denial? I doubt if anyone can withstand these sorts of pressures when they follow a childhood experience filled with emotional difficulties and deceits. Few, if any, normal stable adults can withstand a determined and prolonged attempt at brainwashing, and will ultimately break down. And brainwashing is a minor assault on the mind compared with the sort that parents can mount over the lifetime of a child.

Laing's theories were at first rejected by conventional psychiatry, but now he is getting some support from more academic psychiatrists. His work is of great importance. It shows that the family is responsible for the sanity of its members. It is not simply an individual's bad luck in the genetic card game that leads to his madness, but the tricks of the other players that drive him crazy. When seen from this point of view, "crazy" people, even when their behavior is antisocial, will gain more sympathy.

In his book *The Politics of Experience* Laing says:

> In over 100 cases where we have studied the circumstances around the social event when one person comes to be regarded as schizophrenic, it seems to us that *without exception* the experience and behavior that gets labelled schizophrenic is *a special strategy that a person invents in order to live in an unlivable situation.* In his life situation the person has come to feel he is in an untenable position. He cannot make a move, or make no move, without being beset by contradictory and paradoxical pressures and demands, pushes and pulls, both internally, from himself, and externally, from those around him. He is, as it were, in a position of checkmate.
>
> This state of affairs may not be perceived as such by any of the people in it. The man at the bottom of the heap may be being crushed to death without anyone noticing, much less intending it. The situation here described is impossible to see by studying the different people in it singly. The social system, not single individuals extrapolated from it, must be the object of study.[12]

Laing's theories have had an important influence on therapy. Instead of treating just the individual, some psychiatrists now try to treat the whole family. For example, family crisis therapy operated by Donald G. Langsley and David M. Kaplan at the University of Colorado has been very effective at keeping people out of mental hospitals. Some 60 percent of patients referred for emergency admission to Colorado Psychiatric Hospital, but treated by family therapy instead, were not hospitalized during their breakdown or the following six months. The families are assisted in finding a solution to their own problem, and so in future are more likely to solve the problem themselves than look to the hospital for help.[13]

One case of schizophrenia—that of Daniel Paul Schreber—is perhaps more important than any other single recorded case in psychiatry. Daniel Paul Schreber was analyzed by Freud, who considered him to be the classic case of paranoia. However, a new study of the case made by Dr. Morton Schatzman [14] shows that Schreber's paranoia was almost certainly caused by a repressive regime of child-rearing designed by his father, Dr. Daniel Gottlieb Schreber. This reinterpretation is as valid as was Freud's original analysis, because Freud made his analysis from a published account of Daniel Paul Schreber's illness written by the patient himself in 1903.[15] This document, together with books written by the father about methods of child-rearing, shows how the son Daniel Paul was persecuted and, after a successful career as a distinguished barrister and judge of appeal, eventually went mad. Another of Schreber's sons committed suicide. Yet Schreber himself was venerated for generations in Germany as a "friend of man, children and nature." Two million Germans still belong to Schreber associations dedicated to gymnastics, outdoor pursuits, and allotment gardening.

The importance of the Schreber story lies in the existence of extensive written information from both father and son that shows in detail how the madness of the son resulted from the persecution of the father. It is difficult to believe that such intense relationships as those of the Schreber family would not have had profound effects on the children lasting into later life, or that Schreber's paranoid schizophrenia was simply caused by the development of innate biochemical processes. Study of one individual case cannot by itself justify any generalizations, but one case examined in depth can show how others might be understood.

In classic paranoia as understood by Freud, and by most psychiatrists since, the paranoid person only imagines that he is being persecuted. To label someone as paranoid is to imply that his suffering has no external cause. This conception of paranoia is based on Freud's analysis of Schreber the son. For many years the son suffered from painful and humiliating bodily experiences. He called them "miracles" (*Wunder*) and believed they were performed by God by means of rays. However, these "miracles" were almost certainly psychosomatic symptoms caused by memories of the restrictive leather apparatus that his father compelled him to wear and the exercises he was compelled to perform. The God who performs these miracles in Schreber's fantasies is not difficult to recognize as the sinister Dr. Schreber—the all-powerful God the Father.

Dr. Schreber believed that the bodies of children should be kept straight at all times and in his writings warns parents to fight the child's tendency to sit unevenly, because it deforms the spinal column. He says, "Half resting in lying or wallowing positions should not be allowed. If children are awake they should be alert and hold themselves in straight active positions and be busy." [16] Dr. Schreber recommends that as soon as the sitting child starts to move the back into different positions "the time has come to exchange at least for a few minutes the seated position for an absolutely still supine one." The son describes in his own memoirs what can only be the result of this grueling regime. He cannot acknowledge that his father is to blame for his psychosomatic symptoms in later life, so explains them in terms of divine miracles performed by "rays" (*Strahlen*).

The son suffers from a pain at the base of the spine, which he calls the coccyx miracle. He describes it as "an extremely painful caries-like state of the lowest vertebrae. Its purpose was to make sitting and even lying down impossible. Altogether I was not allowed to remain for long in one and the same position or at the same occupation: when I was walking one attempted to force me to lie down, and when I was lying down wanted to chase me off my bed. Rays did not seem to appreciate at all that a human being who actually exists must be somewhere. . . . I had become an embarrassing being for the rays (for God) in whatever position I might be." [17]

Dr. Schreber devised an ingenious apparatus to prevent restless children from slouching with elbows on the table. The *Geradhalter* (straightholder), available in portable or fixed models, consisted of an iron crossbar fixed rigidly to the table to prevent a child from slouching forward. Dr. Schreber describes in his books testing it on his children. He says that a child could not lean against it for long "because of the pressure of the hard object against the bones and the consequent discomfort." [18] The son describes how in later life he suffered pains in the chest. He writes in his memoirs that "one of the most horrifying of miracles was the so-called compression of the chest miracle" and describes "the oppression caused by lack of breath." [19]

Another piece of apparatus devised by Dr. Schreber was a leather shoulder harness used to strap the child down to the bed to ensure that the child slept on his back in a straight position. He believed that all children should sleep and rest in a straight position lying flat on the back, and expounds in his book *The Harmful Body Positions and Habits of Children* his extraordinary theory that sleeping on the side will impair the nutrition of body tissues on that side, leading to paralysis later in life.

Perhaps the most terrible of Dr. Schreber's tortures were the *Kopfhalter* and chinband. The *Kopfhalter* was attached to the hair at the back of the head and at the other end to the underwear. The purpose was supposed to be to keep the head straight. The son describes in later life headaches that can be seen as vivid memories of the *Kopfhalter*. He writes in his memoirs of "tearing and pulling pains" that were "hardly comparable to ordinary headaches." [20] He describes another miracle that seems to be the result of wearing the chinband, which he refers to obliquely as "the headbinding machine."

These headaches "compressed my head as though in a vise by turning a kind of screw, causing my head to temporarily assume an elongated pear-shaped form." [21]

The father's ideas must have influenced almost every moment of the son's daily life. For the son there was no escape. Dr. Schreber believed that the parent must master the child and the father must rule the family. By all accounts Frau Schreber was a devoted wife, and Dr. Schreber describes the ideal marital relationship like this: "When the man can support his opinions by reason of demonstrable truth, no wife with common sense and goodwill would want to oppose his decisive voice." [22] Although many others in that period may have had the same sort of views, Dr. Schreber was exceptional in being totally obsessed with the idea of controlling his children, to the point where he invented apparatus to subdue them night and day.

Dr. Schreber believed that the freedom of children must be curtailed by harsh disciplines for the sake of their own moral, mental, and physical health. His advice for dealing with a crying child seems today a certain recipe for failure and frustration, leading ultimately to a baby battered emotionally if not physically. He writes:

> One must look at the moods of the little ones which are announced by screaming without reason and crying. . . . If one has convinced oneself that no real need, no disturbing or painful condition, no sickness is present, a mood, a whim, the first appearance of selfwill . . . one has to step forward in a positive manner: by quick distraction of the attention, stern words, threatening gestures, rapping against the bed . . . or when all of this is of no avail—by moderate intermittent, bodily admonishments consistently repeated until the child calms down or falls asleep . . . such a procedure is necessary only once or at most twice and one is master of the child for ever. From now on a glance, a word, a single threatening gesture, is sufficient to rule the child. [23]

This discipline was imposed on every detail of the Schreber children's lives. Nurserymaids and servants were expected to follow the instructions to the letter. Children were not allowed to eat between meals. But nurses were instructed to teach self-restraint by taking a child upon their knees and denying him food while they ate themselves. One nurse was dismissed from service in the Schreber household because she fed a child a slice of pear under such circumstances.

Thousands, if not millions, of Germans must have been tutored according to the theories of the obsessional Dr. Schreber. Daniel Paul Schreber (1842–1911) cannot have been the only one to have been driven mad by his father's educational theories, but few can have suffered as intensely as he did. A philosophy that for some meant only fresh air, cold dips, and firm but cheerful discipline meant for others a terrifying nightmare where any movement of the body might be found to be in error, requiring lengthy corrective punishment. Dr. Schreber is still honored in Germany today through the Schreber Vereine—organizations that promote gardening and fresh-air activities.

The madness of Daniel Paul Schreber can be satisfactorily accounted for by the peculiar preoccupations of his father. It might still be said that the son was somehow susceptible to stress, that perhaps the biochemistry of his brain made him vulnerable to the stresses that he endured. Stronger children might not have gone mad. Can we ask ourselves whether we would not, in Schreber's place, have gone mad as he did? Our answer will simply depend on the artistry with which Schreber's dilemma is presented and whether we can identify with him.

The biochemistry of the brain is important, but in such cases it is difficult to see any reason why it should be the primary cause of madness. Dr. Schatzman writes: "Nearly everyone who has studied families of people called schizophrenic agrees that the irrationality of the schizophrenic finds its rationality in the context of his first family." [24]

Freud and others since have assumed that the paranoid person invents the "conspiracy" against him, but the case of the Schreber family shows how the paranoid person may be a victim of real childhood terror. This terror can be applied by such subtle means that its source is impossible for someone outside the family to recognize, or so bizarre—as in the Schreber case—that it is difficult to believe. The Schreber case is particularly bizarre, but similar stresses and strains may be imposed upon children and adults by verbal discipline and emotional control. The paranoid person may know that a real conspiracy does exist against him, and his problem is to be able to understand it and explain it to others. Emphasis on biochemical and hereditary theories of mental illness makes it more difficult than ever for the personal story of the patient to be understood on its merits.

There is no strong evidence to suggest that manic-depressive psychosis—the only other commonly recognized severe mental illness—is inherited. This mental illness takes two forms: mania and melancholy. When a person is suffering from mania he (or she) is endlessly busy; he may never stop talking, he is full of ideas but never executes them fully because he always becomes involved in the next task. In contrast the melancholic person is profoundly depressed, perhaps to the point of mute immobility. In both states the person is the victim of his hopelessly confused emotions. Identical twins are not always both affected by the illness, so there must be some important environmental factor involved. Hereditarians since Rüdin in 1923 have suggested that manic-depressive psychosis is inherited but have failed to produce any compelling data.[25]

Neuroses—the relatively mild mental disturbances verging on normality—are said by Eysenck to be inherited. Eysenck and Prell write: "Neuroticism . . . constitutes a biological unit which is inherited as a whole." [26] However, another psychologist, Duncan Blewett, attempted to repeat Eysenck and Prell's experiments on another series of twins (assembled by Shields) and was unable to find the same results.[27] Neurosis is often said to be hereditary, but there is absolutely no compelling scientific evidence to suggest this at present. Furthermore, studies of identical twins who often do not share their neuroses suggest that there is a strong environmental influence in neurosis, whether or not there is any hereditary influence.[28]

The dispute about the causes of mental illness is important because entangled in it lies human beings' concept of themselves. If the psychiatrists who look for the cause of mental illness in poor human relationships are right, human nature, or at least personality, is much more fluid and sensitive to influence than many people might care to think.

The idea that personality has this fluidity is uncomfortable for two reasons. First, it tells us all that our own sanity cannot be taken for granted: if we had to endure the stresses and strains endured by schizophrenics many of us would go crazy too. Second, it reminds us that we are all our brother's keeper. We have the power to tip the scales: we can either help to preserve our neighbor's fragile sanity or help to break it.

Another reason why understanding the causes of mental illness is so important is that the two hereditarian and environmental theories imply such different approaches to treatment. If the cause is genetic, then there is hope that a special diet or drug may cure it. But if the principal cause is a failure in relationships within the family, then no drug or diet can do more than treat the symptoms: the basic underlying cause will remain untreated. If the cause does lie in family life, then treatment may perhaps proceed best if the whole family becomes the focus for therapy or if the patient is removed from the family into some other sheltered environment. If madness is learned, there seems no reason why in many cases it cannot be unlearned, given sufficient time and help.

INTELLIGENCE

A person's greatest chance in life comes before he or she ever goes to school. A baby learns to understand language and to speak from its parents, and this understanding forms the basis of learning in school. If the parents have a poor understanding of language or do not talk to the child, then the child cannot learn, however bright it is. A mass of mathematical theorizing by hereditarians such as Jensen, Herrnstein, and Eysenck has obscured this basic fact, promoting a dogma that intelligence is 80 percent inherited. This dogma is based on a tissue of dubious assumptions and inconclusive observations. The hereditarian theory of intelligence has found favor with political conservatives, and as a result children from minority racial and cultural groups, and children with deprived backgrounds, have been denied the second chance they could have. This is the great brain robbery.

CHAPTER 15

Hereditarians and IQ:
The Great Brain Robbery

The first attempts to measure intelligence were made at the beginning of the century by French psychologists Binet and Simon when the French minister of public instruction appointed a commission to study the education of mentally defective children in Paris. Ever since, psychologists have quarreled bitterly over the extent to which measured intelligence is influenced by heredity and the environment. Binet's own views on this were clear, although they are seldom quoted. In 1909 he wrote:

> Some recent philosophers appear to have given their moral support to the deplorable verdict that the intelligence of an individual is a fixed quantity. . . . We must protest at this brutal pessimism. . . . A child's mind is like a field for which an expert farmer has advised a change in the method of cultivating, with the result that in place of a desert land, we now have a harvest. It is in this particular sense that we say that the intelligence of children may be increased. One increases that which constitutes the intelligence of a school child, namely, the capacity to learn.[1]

In Britain, Binet's ideas were taken up by Francis Galton and his pupil Cyril Burt, and from then on the measurement of IQ became inextricably mixed up with the ideas of eugenics. Binet's IQ test provided Galton with a tool he had spent many years preparing for. Galton wrote in his study of hereditary genius in 1869: "I propose to show in this book that man's natural abilities are derived from inheritance, under exactly the same limitations as are the form and physical features of the whole organic world."[2] Galton pursued this idea by examining the pedigree of eminent men in law, literature, science, classical scholarship, and the Church. He found that 80 percent of the relatives of those who had held office as lord chancellor between 1660 and 1865 and 36 percent of high court judges over the same period were also eminent. Overall, Galton found that 31 percent of illustrious men had eminent fathers and 48 percent had eminent sons. He concluded that outstanding ability was inherited.

No scientists today would feel justified in drawing this conclusion from the same data. In Victorian England, as in earlier periods, people were often selected for the professions on the basis of family connections, so Galton's results may merely be taken as showing the high degree of nepotism in England during that period. No doubt there was a hereditary aristocracy of talent, but only because middle-class, privately educated boys got the best education and privileged entry into the universities and professions. Galton did not include among his eminent men the successful manufacturers and businessmen who were at that time making Britain one of the world's richest nations. He also almost totally ignored home environment, early training, and education. To allow for such influences would have acknowledged the possibility that there might be undeveloped sources of ability in society that were thwarted by unfavorable social circumstances and lack of education.

The reason Galton took this extreme hereditarian view of society was in large part because of his intellectual and perhaps even religious commitment to the ideas of his cousin Charles Darwin, author of *The Origin of Species*. Galton wanted to show that the theory of evolution by natural selection applied to human nature as well as to animals and plants. But his book *Hereditary Genius* was also a defense of the establishment as it existed in 1870. The upper classes must have gained great comfort from being told of their intellectual superiority by so distinguished a scientist. As with the recent works of Jensen and Eysenck, it was a scientific defense of the status quo.

Galton made many of his prejudices clear in his writings. For example, he said in his book *Hereditary Genius:* "It is in the most unqualified manner that I object to pretensions of natural equality." Galton saw emigration to the colonies as a means of cleaning up the country: "England has certainly got rid of a great deal of refuse through means of emigration." He also makes it clear in *Hereditary Genius* what he thinks of other races: "The mistakes the negroes made in their own matters were so childish, stupid and simpleton-like, as frequently to make me ashamed of my own species." [3] Galton believed that each class and race had its place and an inevitable fate determined by heredity.

After the entry of the United States into the First World War in 1917, the U.S. Army made great use of IQ tests. Lewis M. Terman, a country schoolmaster who studied at Stanford University, translated and revised the Binet test. After testing and standardizing his version on 2,300 schoolchildren, he published the Stanford-Binet test in 1916.[4]

About the same time, the psychologist R. M. Yerkes organized a highly efficient corps of psychologists to help the American military authorities select personnel. They devised new tests to identify the mentally incompetent and to grade recruits according to ability. Men with low intelligence were either discharged or drafted into units engaged in manual labor. Incompetent officers were discharged or given simple tasks, and competent officers were selected for further training and responsibility. During the war period 1,750,000 men were tested, 8,000 discharged, 10,000 sent to laboring battalions, and 10,000 selected for special training. Yerkes published the results of this work in 1921 in *Psychological Testing in the U.S. Army,* which served as a model for others who wished to make use of IQ testing. Following this example, psychologists were employed by governments to advise about education and to assist with selection for the civil service.[5]

In England, Cyril Burt, who had earlier worked with Galton, was appointed as the first school psychologist to the London County Council. He was the first full-time educational psychologist in Great Britain. It was Burt who first developed the written IQ test with Yes/No answers, and he also developed special tests for educational attainment in reading, spelling, composition, and arithmetic. He set an approach to education testing and selection that was to last for more than half a century. Despite its intellectual brilliance, this approach was colored by Galton's social philosophy. The idea that intelligence was fixed by heredity and remained more or less constant throughout life became popular. Ever since, psychologists have been divided roughly into two camps: the hereditarians and the environmentalists.

There are now many different kinds of IQ tests. Some are designed to estimate the ability of people to use language and numbers; others test understanding of relationships between objects in two and three dimensions or the logical relationships of abstract symbols. When these tests are given to a large number of people it is found that a person who does well in one test is more than likely to do well in another. This is taken by many psychologists to imply that there is a basic ability called *g*—the general ability factor—which various IQ tests measure to a greater or lesser degree. But it is a moot point whether the concept of a basic general intelligence is a valid one. It may be better simply to think of IQ tests in an empirical way as a measurement of a certain kind of ability that psychologists understand and value. The philosopher John Stuart Mill pinpointed the psychologist's dilemma when he said, "The tendency has always been strong to believe that whatever received a name must be an entity of being, having an independent existence of its own. And if no real entity answering to the name could be found, men did not for that reason suppose that none existed, but imagined that it was something peculiarly abstruse and mysterious." [6]

In most IQ tests, the figure 100 has been arbitrarily chosen as a reference point so that people with an IQ score above 100 are above-average in "intelligence" and those below 100 are below-average. Since IQ test results are distributed on a bell-shaped curve in a similar way to height or weight, 50 percent of a typical sample of people will have an IQ above average and 50 percent will have an IQ below average. A little over two thirds of people have IQs between 85 and 115, and 99.7 percent of people have IQs between 55 and 145.

In fact, IQ is not quite distributed according to a mathematically perfect bell-shaped curve. There are more people with low IQs and more people with high IQs than might be expected. Those with IQs below about 50, often known as imbeciles, suffer from severe mental defect resulting from brain damage. This brain damage is caused by accident, disease, or inherited defects such as mongolism that are so severe that they override the effects of the other genes in the individual's constitution.

The brothers and sisters of imbeciles by and large have normal intelligence, which shows that imbecility is not an extreme example of low intelligence but an exceptional occurrence resulting from chance genetic or environmental processes. The brothers and sisters of "feeble-minded" persons with IQs in the range of 50 to 75, on the other hand, have a lower intelligence than the brothers and sisters of imbeciles, which shows that feeble-mindedness is not a chance occurrence but tends to recur in families. It may sometimes be caused by hereditary factors but can also be caused by an impoverished environment. The parents of severely subnormal children come from all strata of society, whereas the parents of feeble-minded children come predominantly from the lower social classes. Indeed, mild subnormality without sign of damage to the nervous system is virtually confined to poor families. The cause is almost certainly the lack of stimulation and opportunity to learn when living conditions are poor and the parents themselves come from a deprived background and so, without help, have little to offer their own children.

There is another bulge in the "normal" distribution curve of IQ scores between 70 and 90. This is often explained as the result of individual scores being depressed by temporary environmental disadvantages and emotional factors. Indeed, Cyril Burt found that when the test scores of subjects who had suffered emotional upsets at the time of testing were removed from the distribution the bulge disappeared. If these subjects are retested later, the IQs of many of them are found to have increased.

The excess of gifted people found at the top end of the IQ range has been explained in several ways. Burt has suggested that there may be major genes that affect intellectual abilities in the same way that other major genes cause abnormality. However, there is no direct evidence for the existence of such genes. Another suggestion is that highly intelligent men marry highly intelligent women and so have children who, because they have better opportunities to learn, become superintelligent. It is also possible that the bulge at the top end of the IQ range is the result of highly gifted people creating an environment for themselves in which they have the opportunity to develop their intelligence much further than the average.

There are genes that cause severe mental retardation and low IQ. However, these genes are rare and so have no real effect on the overall distribution of IQ in the population as a whole. No genes are known that actually lead to an increased performance of the brain. If genius is hereditary, it is certainly not inherited as a simple gene, such as the genes causing phenylketonuria or red hair. The hereditary influence on intelligence is almost certainly caused by many genes, all of which have a small effect in themselves. Each of these genes has such a small individual effect that it cannot be recognized. There is no direct evidence that these genes exist. They are theoretical and have been proposed simply to explain the observation that IQ is partly inherited.

Genes must undoubtedly exist that control the structure and function of the brain, just as blueprints exist that specify the design of a computer. These blueprints are quite different from the computer program, which tells the computer how to operate at any particular moment. The range and versatility of the programs available to a computer can be compared with the range and versatility of a person's intelligence. The performance of a computer is as good as its program; so it is with the human brain. However, the program of the human brain is, at least in large measure, assembled through experience of the environment and opportunities available for learning. An inferior computer or a damaged brain may perform better than a superior computer or brain if it has been better programmed.

In the late 1960s, following President Johnson's Anti-Poverty Bill, many attempts were made to improve the environment of poor and deprived children in the United States. The hope was that this would improve the intelligence of these children and give them a better chance in life. Millions of dollars were spent on the Headstart program, with the aim of improving the education of negroes and underprivileged people. The hope was that a few hours' extra teaching a week would make an impression on children despite years of neglect. But Headstart did not live up to its expectations. An official evaluation of Headstart made by the Westinghouse Learning Corporation in 1969 showed that the full-year Headstart program did have a positive effect on increasing readiness for school and language ability, but the effects were small. The short summer Headstart program had no effect.[7] However, some more intensive compensatory education programs that begin with younger children are now proving to be successful.[8]

Eager to find respectable reasons for the failure of Headstart, some educational psychologists have chosen to blame the negro himself for his innate shortcomings in intelligence. "Compensatory education has been tried and it has failed," wrote Arthur Jensen in 1969.[9] It was the first sentence of a learned paper published in the *Harvard Educational Review* that triggered a major controversy about the inheritance of intelligence.

Jensen argues that since progress in compensatory education programs is usually measured by changes in the IQs of the pupils, the success of such programs may be forecast from a knowledge of the way in which IQ is inherited. If disadvantaged children have low IQs because of their inherited constitution rather than their poor circumstances, it is a waste of time trying to improve their intelligence by the usual compensatory programs. He also urges a new approach to the teaching of disadvantaged children based on his theory that these children learn best by rote.

Jensen's article created a public furor and was rapidly exploited by whites in the Deep South of the United States, where the article was taken to support the belief that "white teachers could not understand the nigra mind'' and was used to oppose school integration. Martin Deutsch, professor of early childhood education at New York University, commented: "I believe the impact of Jensen's article was destructive; that it has had negative implications for the struggle against racism and for the improvement of the educational system. The conclusions he draws are, I believe, unwarranted by the existing data, and reflect a consistent bias towards a racist hypothesis." [10] In Britain, Jensen's arguments were given support and publicity by Hans Eysenck, particularly in two books, *Race, Intelligence and Education* [11] and *The Inequality of Man*. [12] Eysenck has always denied accusations of racism. He has been at pains to point out that he has never said that colored people as a whole—as opposed to American negroes—are innately inferior in intelligence to American whites. However, Eysenck does begin to extend his argument of inherited inferior IQ to other "coloreds," such as Australian aborigines.

Although I am not suggesting that Jensen and Eysenck had any political motive in publishing their studies, the effect has been to lend support to the segregationist case in the United States and South Africa. Jensen himself has strongly protested that he is in favor of integration of the races in schools and of treating each person, black or white, on his or her individual merits. He has testified to this effect before congressional committees. However, he is opposed to compensatory education for deprived and backward children and would like to see these children taught more by rote.

Jensen's thesis was hedged about with so many qualifications that there was bound to be confusion about what he was trying to say. This, for example, is his major conclusion:

> . . . all we are left with are various lines of evidence, no one of which is definitive alone, but which, viewed altogether, make it a not unreasonable hypothesis that genetic factors are strongly implicated in the average Negro-white intelligence difference. The preponderance of evidence is, in my opinion, less consistent with a strictly environmental hypothesis than with a genetic hypothesis, which, of course, does not exclude the influence of environment on its interaction with genetic factors. [13]

Most people will find nothing to disagree with in this statement: it has so many disclaimers it succeeds in saying nothing. Richard C. Lewontin, professor of biology at the University of Chicago, commented: "To contrast a 'strictly environmental hypothesis' with 'a genetic hypothesis which does not exclude the influence of the environment' is to be guilty of the utmost triviality." [14]

Jensen obviously wants to have it both ways. He is trying to say something positive and at the same time, in effect, disclaiming that he has said it. Lewontin goes on to translate the passage like this: "It is pretty clear, although not absolutely proved, that most of the difference in IQ between blacks and whites is genetical." [15] Put even more bluntly, if Jensen is saying anything at all he is saying that blacks in the United States are innately inferior to the whites in IQ. Jensen is careful not to generalize about blacks and whites outside the United States, since there is relatively little relevant data, and blacks in the United States are obviously not a random sample of African blacks.

The basis of the Jensen-Eysenck race theory is that intelligence is 80 percent inherited. Eysenck says: "One important reason for the existence and composition of the 'Lumpenproletariat' may be the genetically determined low intelligence of many of those who have descended into it." He also points out that the Irish have a lower intelligence than the English and the average American white. This is explained by the theory that "over many centuries the most able and adventurous of citizens" have been drawn away to other countries. But he admits that "if we compared negroes with Irish whites, we would conclude that whites and blacks had identical IQs." [16]

Eysenck's suggestion that it was the most intelligent whites who emigrated from Ireland has been repeatedly attacked as historically naïve, and Eysenck has more recently offered another explanation. He suggests that the most intelligent Irishmen enter the priesthood, where they remain celibate and so do not pass on their genes to later generations. An alternative explanation, not considered by Eysenck, is that the predominantly rural culture of Southern Ireland emphasizes the acquisition of skills other than those measured by intelligence tests.

No one seriously disputes the fact that the intelligence of various races and social classes, measured by available IQ tests, does differ. The IQ of U.S. negroes has repeatedly been found to be *on average* fifteen to twenty points lower than that of U.S. whites. It is quite another matter, however, to argue that these differences are largely inherited. Study of the inheritance of IQ can only be done indirectly on large numbers of people using a technical measurement, known as heritability. The theory of heritability has been thoroughly worked out by geneticists and verified with studies of fruit flies and other animals, but useful application of the theory to man has always been very difficult, if not impossible. Dr. Jerry Hirsch, a scientist who specializes in the genetics of behavior, has said, "The plain facts are that in the study of man a heritability estimate turns out to be a piece of knowledge that is both deceptive and trivial." [17]

Heritability is a measure of the proportion of variation in a characteristic that is influenced by genes. In people this measure can only be arrived at indirectly because, unlike animals, people cannot be submitted to breeding experiments. The heritability of animals can be measured accurately. Farmers and stockbreeders find these measurements useful because they tell them how effective they can expect a particular breeding program to be. When the heritability of a characteristic is zero, the variation in the characteristic is considered to be caused entirely by the environment, and when the heritability is 100 percent, then variation in the character is considered to be caused entirely by heredity. For example, the heritability of butterfat content in cows' milk has been found in one series of observations to be 60 percent, whereas heritability of total milk yield has been found to be only 30 percent. This tells the breeder that he will more easily be able to breed cows that produce milk with high butterfat content than cows that produce more milk—at least using that particular farming method. If the farmer were to change his method of farming, then the heritabilities could change radically. Since the measurement of heritability is made in one particular environment, the animal breeder who plans his breeding program on the basis of calculations made in another environment could go wrong. Nor would the same value for heritability necessarily be obtained from two different breeds of cattle kept under identical environmental conditions. Similarly, there is no reason to believe that a value for heritability of IQ calculated in one group of people will apply to other groups of people living in other conditions.

Eysenck's popularization of Jensen's theories does not look into the basic genetic evidence for arriving at the 80 percent figure for heritability of IQ. Eysenck says, "The evidence is well enough known to be mentioned only in passing." [18] He is content to accept Jensen's estimates of heritability at face value. And Jensen himself makes sweeping claims that "the heritability of the IQ . . . comes out at about 80 percent, the average value obtained from *all the relevant studies now reported*" (my italics). [19] However, new doubt has now been cast on Jensen's calculations of heritability by Christopher Jencks and colleagues at the Center for Educational Policy Research at Harvard University. [20] By lumping a large number of different studies together to produce one magical figure, Jensen has overlooked the fact that different methods of calculating heritability and different sets of data produce quite different answers. The same error has been repeated by Eysenck. A devastating analysis by Leon J. Karmin (*The Science and Politics of I.Q.*, New York: John Wiley, 1974) of the data on which Jensen's thesis is based shows additional fundamental errors.

Measures of heritability say nothing about what will happen following some improvement in the environment. Indeed, they assume that the environment is unchanging. But new environmental influences may arise that make all previous measurements of heritability invalid. Conventional measures of heritability for human height, for example, have values of about 80 to 100 percent, which suggests that heredity has a very great influence on variation in height—at least at the time when heritability was calculated. Since then the average height of people in both America and Japan has increased spectacularly as a result of unidentified changes in the environment. This would not have been predicted from knowledge of heritability of height. The only real use to which measures of human heritability can be put is to make them the basis for a eugenic breeding program. Perhaps this is what some scientists who take the hereditarian view are ultimately aiming for.

Indeed, Jensen has asked a rhetorical question that reflects this type of eugenic approach: "Is there a danger that current welfare policies, unaided by eugenic foresight, could lead to the genetic enslavement of a substantial segment of our population?" and has answered it by saying that "differential birth rates in the population that are correlated with educationally and occupationally relevant traits of high heritability could produce long term dysgenic trends which would make environmental amelioration of the plight of the disadvantaged increasingly difficult." [21]

This extraordinary sentence might be translated as follows: People with inferior intelligence have larger families than those with normal intelligence. Intelligence is largely inherited: therefore the long-term trend will be harmful to the evolution of the human species. It will become increasingly difficult to ameliorate the plight of these people by altering the environment. (*Dysgenic* means tending to be harmful to the hereditary qualities or evolution of the human species.) Referring back to Jensen's original rhetorical question, he appears to be suggesting that present welfare policies will make the plight of the disadvantaged worse in future unless they are based on eugenic principles. In effect, Jensen seems to be calling for the distribution of welfare not according to people's real needs but according to their desirability as breeding stock.

Such a breeding program would simply increase the deprivation of those people who are already badly off and penalize them and their children further. Their environment would deteriorate, and so would their IQs. The Jensen-Eysenck argument grossly underestimates the importance of environment.

The average IQ of twins seems to be about five points lower than the average IQ of people born singly. This difference has been studied by R. G. Record, Thomas McKeown, and J. H. Edwards of Birmingham University, England, who found that the difference could not be explained by differences in the age of the mothers, the birth order or birth weight, or other prenatal influences. They went on to investigate the IQs of 148 twins whose co-twins were stillborn or died within four weeks of birth. They found that their IQs were only a little lower than the IQs of people born singly.[22] This suggests that the divided attention twins get from parents and others has an appreciable effect on the twins' IQ. Twins have been found in several studies to lag behind other children in talking and skill with words. This is probably also because they tend to communicate a lot with each other nonverbally. This effect of environment amounts to only five IQ points. This type of environmental influence could account for a large part of the average difference in IQ of blacks and whites and people in different social classes. In Israel, for example, Jewish children of European origin have average IQs of 105 and Jewish children of Middle Eastern origin brought up at home have IQs of only 85—near Jensen's danger point. However, when these children are raised in a kibbutz on the same nursery training schedule, both lots of children have the same average IQ of 115. This extreme change in home environment adds an average of 30 IQ points to the intelligence of Middle Eastern Jewish children.[23] Children who are genetically well endowed with IQ are often born into favorable environments. Parents with genes favoring high IQ tend to provide unusually rich home environments, regardless of whether the children also have genes favoring high intelligence. Therefore some children have a double advantage. They have the most favorable genes and the most favorable environments. Conversely, other children have a double disadvantage. Some children who are not particularly well endowed with genes for IQ nevertheless benefit from the favorable environment provided by intelligent parents. This special advantage (technically known as the covariance) of being born to intelligent parents normally accounts for about 20 percent of IQ scores.

Since heritability may vary with race and environment, it must be separately measured for each race and environment. And because of the segregation of negroes both physically and socially in the United

States, it is quite unrealistic to assume that heritability of IQ would be the same for both negroes and whites.

Nevertheless, Jensen argues that genetic differences in IQ between blacks and whites are evident when blacks and whites with the same socioeconomic status are compared. For this purpose he defines socio-economic status in terms of occupation, schooling, and income. These are genuine measures of the quality of the environment but can still be misleading. Negroes go to poorer schools than whites, so even if they have stayed at school for the same length of time they will not have had the same opportunities to acquire IQ. Within a given type of oc-cupation there are large differences in ability and it would generally be expected that within a given occupation the negroes would be in the lower level because of their initial disadvantages and because of preju-dice. Similarly with income: there are many advantages which money cannot buy.

So what are the facts about inheritance of IQ? There is no doubt that there is a hereditary effect on IQ, but it is impossible to measure it exactly because it seems to vary with the type of environment. What the figures do show is that environment has a large effect on IQ in both British and American society. The effect of environment on vari-ations in IQ in a group of people is probably as great as the effect of heredity, and may be greater. Jensen and Eysenck have failed to take into account the special interaction of heredity with environment: their calculations were made on the assumption that this factor was rather small and scarcely worth bothering about. It is therefore ironic that Eysenck claims to be an "interactionist" and says that the hereditarian position is an interactionist position. Jensen also neglects interaction when he studies the environment to find single environmental factors affecting IQ. Environmental factors interact with each other and may multiply each other—these interactions must be studied before the ef-fects of the environment can be fully accounted for.

Eysenck believes that "all the evidence to date suggests the strong and indeed overwhelming importance of genetic factors in producing the great variety of intellectual differences which we observe in our culture, and much of the difference observed between certain racial groups." [24] As far as Eysenck is concerned, there appears to be little hope for the U.S. negro. Like Jensen, he does not believe that com-pensatory education will provide the answer, because even if it does work it will be too expensive. However, when the experimental phase of compensatory education is over, methods may be found of provid-ing it much more cheaply. And if the cost is regarded as an investment and deducted from the cost of maintaining inadequate children and families in institutions it will not appear so expensive.

Since Jensen wrote his article a number of experts have been willing to come forward and criticize the theory. Two distinguished geneticists, Professor Walter F. Bodmer and Professor Luigi Cavalli-Sforza, are among the scientists who have repudiated Jensen and Eysenck. They wrote in an article in *Scientific American:* "As geneticists, we can state with certainty that there is no *a priori* reason why genes affecting IQ . . . should be such that on average whites have significantly more genes increasing IQ than blacks do." [25]

Cambridge geneticist Professor J. M. Thoday has pointed out important weaknesses in Jensen's argument. He writes: "Jensen suffers from the same kind of conscious or unconscious bias as many of his opponents, that is to say he is prepared to accept evidence that seems to support his hypothesis with less critical examination than he would give to evidence purporting to be against him." [26] Thoday gives two examples of bias in Jensen's arguments—here I shall only mention one.

Jensen claims that the phenomenon known to statisticians as "regression to the mean" is predictable from genetic considerations and is therefore evidence supporting his hypothesis that IQ is 80 percent hereditary. Eysenck puts forward a similar argument in his book *The Inequality of Man*. To illustrate what is meant by "regression to the mean" in relation to IQ, consider a group of people with an average IQ of 120. The average IQ of their children will be about 108. And if a group of people have an average IQ of 80, their children should have an average IQ of 92. It is a simple observation that the average IQ of the children in each case has "regressed toward the mean" IQ of 100. Jensen supports his case with evidence that the IQ of whites regresses toward the average white IQ of 100 while the IQ of blacks regresses toward the average for U.S. blacks of 80. Thoday says: "Jensen regards this evidence as supporting the genetic hypothesis. For some time I fell into the same trap. But it is a trap, for populations must regress to their own mean whatever the cause, genetic or environmental, of the mean differences between populations." [27]

The Jensen-Eysenck theory of race and IQ can only be called the Great Brain Robbery. There has never been sufficient hard scientific evidence to warrant a theory of this kind, which points an accusing finger at all black people in the United States and by implication at black people everywhere. Collectively black Americans have been judged by Jensen and Eysenck to be innately inferior in intelligence.

This judgment has been given spurious authority by the claim that 90 percent of all experts agree with it. Irishmen and Australian aborigines have suffered a similar slur. The theory has reinforced existing prejudices that blacks as a whole are inferior.

The terrible consequence of this type of theory is that it can be self-fulfilling. When failure is expected, it often comes. Whether the theory is true or not, if sufficient people believe in it, it might become true. The energetic promotion of this theory has already held up the provision of better teaching for blacks and other minority groups in the United States and has provided a convenient theoretical bolster for repressive educational practices in South Africa. The consequence is that colored people are being robbed of the opportunity to develop their brains. Other minority groups such as Mexicans and Puerto Ricans in the United States and Irish and West Indians in Britain are similarly categorized and robbed of opportunity, although these minority groups have been much less well studied.

CHAPTER 16

Professor Shockley and His
Thinking Exercises

"When life gives you lemons, make lemonade." This is the cheerful philosophy of Professor William Shockley, who gave the world the transistor and was rewarded in 1956 with the Nobel Prize—the highest honor in science. Professor Shockley is one expert who has given both Jensen and Eysenck unqualified support. Shockley is a physicist, but he has made use of the theories of Jensen and Eysenck on the genetic causes of low intelligence and criminality to support a long campaign publicizing his belief that most negroes have an inherited low intelligence. Or—as Professor Shockley would probably prefer to put it—this is the opinion to which his research inescapably leads. Professor Shockley is worried that people with low intelligence, particularly blacks, will breed faster than whites with high intelligence and so the quality of the human species in the United States will deteriorate.

Professor Shockley is an expert in ferromagnetism, the properties of metals, and the theory of solids, none of which has the remotest connection with human genetics, but he became interested in the race-IQ question after reading the story of Rudy Hoskins, "the Brute," in the *San Francisco Chronicle*. Here Shockley himself takes up the story:

> Blinding acid in the eyes of San Francisco delicatessen proprietor Harry Goldman thrown from a baby bottle by a teenager Rudy Hoskins was the 1963 news story that was probably more influential than any other single cause in initiating my active concern with the possible dysgenic [i.e., anti-evolutionary] effects of modern society. Rudy Hoskins, nicknamed "the Brute", had an IQ of 60 to 65 and was one of 17 illegitimate children of a woman reported to have an IQ of 55, who could remember

the names of only nine of her children. Is she an isolated statistic? Who knows? For myself, I fear it is not an isolated statistic. I can see how if this sort of thing can occur at all in our society, it could snowball so that the fraction of our population composed of such people could double in less than 20 years and outnumber all others in a few centuries. Obviously, any substantial percentage of people like this could produce enormous social instability. . . .[1]

Shockley's campaign to bring his version of scientific truth to other scientists and the public is an extraordinary tale of one man's single-mindedness—the sort of single-mindedness that must have been a great advantage to him when he was working on the transistor at Bell Telephone Laboratories. Shockley, armed with his Nobel Laureate, has worked hard to attract the attention of both the public and the academic world to his belief that criminals, the insane, and those with low intelligence are breeding so fast that they are reducing the genetic quality of the white race in the United States and threatening to swamp it. His ideas are based on a revamped version of the bad-heredity concept that predates modern genetics. Shockley denies that he is a racist. However, he has an almost mystical obsession with the hereditary potential of races. For example, he said in a talk read to the National Academy of Sciences in the spring of 1968, "The basis for human civilization is concern for memories of emotions stored in neurological systems of earth's hereditary sequence." [2] This is one of two postulates considered by Shockley to be fundamental for civilized men. Although the statement uses scientific terminology, it is simply a personal declaration of Shockley's mysticism, which has more in common with the God-was-an-astronaut school of thought than with academic science.

Many of Shockley's arguments are based on the theories of Jensen and Eysenck. For example, he is impressed by Eysenck's theory that neurosis and extroversion are largely inherited. He notes that unmarried mothers and women prisoners are more neurotic and extrovert than average and then asks the question: "Can it mean that unwed mothers do on average transmit genetically controlled behavior traits that predispose the children to becoming prisoners?" Shockley says he finds it hard to reject "the whole concept of bad heredity conveyed by Eysenck's findings." [3] Jensen's theories of intelligence and race are even more central to Shockley's arguments, and Shockley has campaigned vigorously to bring Jensen's theories to a wide audience. Until Jensen and Eysenck take measures to disentangle themselves from Shockley, the ideas of these three men must remain closely associated.

Jensen feeds Shockley and Shockley feeds the racialists—people who are impatient about making significant investment to improve the conditions of the blacks and who would welcome any excuse to be off loaded with it.

Since taking up the cause of eugenics, Shockley has been accident-prone. Talks scheduled to be given by him have been canceled at the last moment, his requests that funds be allocated to investigate the question have been turned down, and Leeds University in England at the last moment decided not to confer on him an honorary doctorate. What is it about Shockley that stirs up greater passions than even Jensen or Eysenck arouse? Shockley is ambivalent and his writings often obscure, but they do show that he is prepared to go at least one stage further than Jensen or Eysenck. Shockley talks explicitly about the sterilization of people with "bad heredity." He does not actually advocate this in so many words, but recommends that we use it as a "thinking exercise." For example, here is a thinking exercise of Shockley's designed to familiarize the student with the "deci-child certificate plan."

> Here is the plan divided into five steps: Step 1: The public votes for the rate of population increase, say one third per cent per year so that population will double in two centuries. Step 2: The Census Bureau computes that this means on the average 2.2 children per each girl that reaches maturity. Step 3: The public health agencies ensure that every girl becomes sterile by subcutaneous injection, at an early age, of the time capsule. The time capsule is a small silicon sponge providing a slow seepage of the contraceptive hormone being developed by Dr. Sheldon Segal, the population council's biomedical research director. She will then remain sterile until the sponge is removed. Step 4: Upon reaching maturity every girl is issued with 22 deci-child certificates. A married couple could use 10 of these to pay for sponge removal until after birth of a child. Then a new time capsule is installed. Step 5: After two babies, the couple can either sell the remaining two deci-child certificates through any member firm of the New York Stock Exchange or buy eight more on the open market and have a third pregnancy. In fact, a girl intending to become a nun could sell her certificates immediately upon their receipt.[4]

Shockley sees the main consequence of the time capsule plus deci-child certificate plan as allowing only those people who want children and can afford them to continue to have them.

Although Shockley insists that these and other proposals are only thinking exercises rather than plans for action, we are presumably supposed to take them seriously. If this proposal could be put into effect, which seems most unlikely in our present society, children would become a stock market commodity most easily available to those with most money. Shockley presumably hopes that the better off would then have proportionately more children than the less well off, and so human genetic quality would improve. But there is no real evidence to suggest that the wealthy will make the best parents. And if the wealthy have larger families, the average intelligence of their children may well start to decline because each child will get less individual attention. Shockley has also suggested a macabre "thinking exercise" involving brain transplants between different races and sexes. "Can we predict on the basis of known psychological laws, just as Einstein predicted the $E = mc^2$ relationship by applying existing theory to an impossibly demanding conceptual experiment, how the actually impossible conceptual experiment of a brain transplant might alter the mental powers and personality developed by the brain after transplanting it to its new environment? In an intersex or interracial transplant, how would the brain adapt? What facts about transvestites can be used as postulates for such conceptual experiments?"

This thought experiment reads like the scenario for a comic book sequence of Brainiac or the Mad Thinker. These are comic book stereotypes of the mad scientist who works for some evil government and is usually portrayed as a small misshapen man with a large egghead. The brains of these stereotype mad scientists are so accustomed to calculations that they always neglect the human factor, which cannot be expressed in figures. They fail to understand that biology and psychology cannot be reduced to mathematical laws as can physics.

Dr. Frankenstein went further than a brain transplant: he re-created an entire body from its parts. But the one thing he was unable to provide for the new creature was love and human understanding. So the creature went berserk. There is a lesson here.

Another question arising from this macabre thinking exercise is why a brain transplant should be presumed necessary for such a "thinking exercise" when perhaps a skin transplant would do? A skin transplant would at least serve as a useful scientific comparison. Such surgery, if possible, would allow a test to be made of the effect of a change of skin color alone on a person's life. But surgery is not necessary: white skins can be made black and black skins white if one is prepared to take drugs. John Howard Griffin described his experiences of changing the color of his skin from white to black in his book *Black*

Like Me. He discovered the horror of being black in a world of hostile whites.

Griffin's experience alone is insufficient to provide scientifically valid conclusions, but his experience is valid. There is no reason why Griffin's experiment should not be repeated by others on a scale large enough to assess the results scientifically. This is how Griffin felt when suddenly he had a black skin in the Southern states of America:

> I walked through the streets of Mobile throughout the afternoon. I had known the city before, in my youth, when I sailed from there once to France. I knew it then as a privileged white. It had impressed me as a beautiful Southern port town, gracious and calm. I had seen the Negro dock workers stripped to the waist, their bodies glistening with sweat under their loads. The sight had chilled me, touched me to pity for men who so resembled beasts of burden. But I had dismissed it as belonging to the natural order of things. The Southern whites I knew were kind and wise. If they allowed this, then surely it must be right.
>
> Now, walking the same streets as a Negro, I found no trace of the Mobile I formerly knew, nothing familiar. The laborers still dragged out their ox-like lives, but the gracious Southerner, the wise Southerner, the kind Southerner, was nowhere visible. I knew that if I were white I would find him easily, for his other face is there for whites to see. It is not a false face; it is simply different from the one the Negro sees. The Negro sees him as a man with muscular emotions who wants to drive out all his race except the beasts of burden. I concluded that, as in everything else, the atmosphere of a place is entirely different for Negro and white. The Negro sees and reacts differently not because he is Negro, but because he is suppressed.

Griffin concluded that skin color alone is the cause of negro "inferiority."

> I have held no brief for the Negro. I have looked for all aspects of "inferiority" among them and I cannot find them. All the cherished question-begging epithets applied to the Negro race, and widely accepted as truth even by men of good will, simply prove untrue when one lives among them. This, of course, excludes the trash element, which is the same everywhere and is no more evident among Negroes than whites. When all the talk, all the propaganda, has been cut away, the criterion is nothing but the color of skin. My experience proved that. They judged me by no other quality. My skin was dark. That was sufficient reason for them to deny me those rights and freedoms without which life loses its significance and becomes a matter of little more than animal survival.
>
> I searched for some answer and found none. I had spent a day without

food and water for no other reason than that my skin was black. I was sitting on a tub in a swamp for no other reason.[5]

But Shockley believes that skin color exists for a purpose. He says: "Nature has color-coded groups of individuals so that statistically reliable predictions of their adaptability to intellectually rewarding and effective lives can easily be made and profitably used by the pragmatic man in the street." [6]

Shockley has taken his campaign to the U.S. National Academy of Sciences and has asked that a study be made of disadvantaged children. One object of the study would be, as Shockley has put it, to answer the question: "Can improved environment remedy the obviously enormous social disadvantages afflicting the illegitimate 25 percent of negro babies?" [7] Shockley's own answer to this question expressed in a letter to the academy and signed by five other scientists—none of whom are geneticists—is: "We believe that irrefutable evidence continues to accumulate for the inheritance of genetically controlled socially maladaptive traits." [8]

Shockley's request for more research funds to look at the race-IQ question was turned down almost unanimously by the U.S. National Academy of Sciences, and in a statement made on October 23, 1967, the council of the academy sounded a note of warning. It said the council "is mindful of the extent to which preliminary or rudimentary facts concerning human genetics can be used to further the goals of those with more than a scientific mission." [9] The statement acknowledges that it would be possible in theory to select a human superrace with high IQ, but that it would be a rather slow and unpredictable process. Then it says:

> It is contrary to all evidence that social problems such as poverty, slums, school dropouts, and crime are entirely genetic. There is surely a substantial and perhaps overriding environmental and social component. Therefore society need not wait for future heredity environment research in order to attempt environmental improvements, nor will it do so.[10]

The academicians also questioned whether it made sense to consider eugenic means of improving society when straightforward measures of population control such as contraception and abortion are still not freely available to all and are still restricted by law. Contraception has only recently been available to many poor people long after it has been available to the well-educated and well-to-do.

Eysenck and Jensen have failed to publicly repudiate Shockley's more extreme ideas. Eysenck refers to "W. Shockley, the Nobel prize winner," in his book *Race, Intelligence and Education.* Eysenck is content to make use of Shockley's prestige without making clear the extraordinary nature of his ideas. Perhaps Shockley is simply an innocent expert who has wandered off the path into unfamiliar territory, misled by his own eminence in another field. Shockley himself says, "I sincerely and thoughtfully believe that my current attempts to demonstrate that American negro shortcomings are preponderantly hereditary is the action most likely to reduce negro agony in future." [11]

CHAPTER 17

Social Engineering:
The IQ Plot Thickens

One day in 1935 two backward babies living in a state orphanage in Iowa were transferred to an institution for the feeble-minded. The younger one, aged thirteen months, had an IQ of 46 and could not stand when given assistance. The older one, aged sixteen months, also with an IQ of 46, could not walk even if assisted and made no attempts to make the usual baby noises. To the authorities who decided to transfer them, there was no doubt that they were feeble-minded. But six months later a psychologist visiting the ward was surprised to see that the two children had developed rapidly. When tested, their IQs were found to have leapt ahead by 31 and 52 points, and at the age of three and a half their IQs were 95 and 93, which is well within the normal range.

The two feeble-minded babies had been placed in a ward with moron girls who had a mental age of from five to nine years. Psychologists H. M. Skeels and H. B. Dye described in 1939 how the moron girls stimulated these two severely retarded babies and—incredibly— increased their intelligence:

> . . . the older brighter girls on the ward became very much attached to the children and would play with them during most of their waking hours. Moreover the attendants on the ward also took a great fancy to the babies, took them with them on their days off, took them to the store, brought them toys, picture books, and play materials. On the basis of this clinical surprise, came the fantastic plan of transferring mentally retarded children, one to two years of age, from the orphanage nursery to an institution for the feeble minded in order to make them normal.[1]

Thirteen retarded children aged seven to thirty months were then transferred to wards of feeble-minded adult girls. Twelve other retarded children with slightly higher IQs were chosen for comparison and were left in the orphanage. Every one of the children transferred to the ward for the feeble-minded showed a steady gain in IQ. The minimum gain was 7 points and the maximum 58 points. Most showed gains of over 20 points. However, the children who were left in the orphanage and were originally more intelligent actually showed a decrease in IQ. This study was severely criticized on statistical grounds when it was first published in 1939, but recently these children were followed up, after a gap of twenty years or more.[2, 3]

All the children in the study were finally traced, except for one who had died. The differences between the two groups when in their twenties could not have been more marked. All of the thirteen in the experimental group who were transferred to the ward for the feeble-minded and looked after by the feeble-minded girls were self-supporting. Eleven were married and nine had children. Of the twelve who had remained in the orphanage, five continued to be wards of state institutions. Seven were employed, three of them as dishwashers and one in a cafeteria, another traveled from coast to coast doing odd jobs, another was an employee in an institution in which he was formerly a patient. Only one of this group had a good job (as a typesetter for a newspaper), a stable marriage, children, and a home of his own. His treatment had been quite different from the other children in his group because he was thought to be deaf and so was transferred to a residential school for the partially deaf. The matron of his cottage took a special interest in him because he was the youngest in the group, and because he had no family he was often a guest in her home. He was the only member of the orphanage group to get beyond the eighth grade, whereas one member of the experimental group went to college and got a B.A. degree, another graduated from business school, and three girls went to college for varying periods.

The jobs of the experimental group were also much better. The three men in the group were a sales manager, a vocational counselor, and a staff sergeant in the air force. Eight out of the ten girls in the group had married. Two were nurses, one was a beautician, and one taught in elementary school.

The enormous difference in the adult fates of these two groups of children was not all a result of the experimental group being transferred from the orphange to the institutions for the feeble-minded. This was just the first stage where they benefited from the care and attention of the feeble-minded girls. After that, the experimental children went to an institution where they had their own foster mothers, and eleven of the thirteen were later adopted. The differences between the adults in the two groups reflect differences between children who have been severely deprived and children who have had a fair chance.

This heroic follow-up made by Skeels and his colleagues shows what a difference early intervention can make to the life of a child. Other studies have shown that when deprived children are given intensive stimulation, IQ scores sometimes go up 20 or 30 points.

Jensen argues that all these cases are exceptional examples of the effect of the environment and that under ordinary circumstances the environment has a very small effect on intelligence within the range calculated from heritability measurements. He introduces the idea of a threshold above which the environment has little effect:

> Below a certain threshold of environmental adequacy, deprivation can have a markedly depressing effect on intelligence. But above this threshold, environmental variations cause relatively small differences in intelligence. The fact that the vast majority of the populations sampled in studies of the heritability of intelligence are above this threshold level of environmental adequacy accounts for high values of the heritability estimates and the relatively small proportion of IQ variance attributable to environmental influences.[4]

This is a convenient ad hoc hypothesis, but why should we believe it when other studies show that permanent gains in IQ can be made by children who are deprived but not to a pathological extent?

IQ may vary throughout life and increase or decrease according to circumstances.

Hereditarians argue that intelligence is, if not altogether constant, at least stable. Indeed, they have no alternative but to argue this if they are to maintain, as they do, that intelligence is largely inherited and little influenced by environment. They point out that when a group of people is retested after a certain period, the IQs as measured in the two tests are strongly correlated. However even high correlations can conceal large individual changes in IQ.

IQ becomes increasingly stable with age because it is dependent upon the accumulation of experience. With increasing age, past experience, as measured by one IQ test, forms an increasing proportion of total experience, which is measured by a second IQ test. Two tests made at, for example, twelve and nine will obviously correlate more highly than two tests made at five and two because a greater common background of experience exists in the tests made at a later age, although the time interval between them is the same.

When individual cases are separated out from the mass of correlations it appears that anything can happen to a person's IQ over a matter of years, although it is likely that if a person remains in a reasonably stable environment his or her IQ is likely to remain stable. Evidence showing that the apparent stability of IQ comes from the stability of the environment can be found in studies of individuals who all had the same measured IQ at an early age. In one study a small group of children with IQs ranging from 96 to 103 at age six were found to have IQs ranging from 90 to 132 when followed up twenty-seven years later. Gifted children, perhaps more than any others, show a wide spread of achievement in later life.

The effects of environment on IQ can also be measured in large groups of people under changing circumstances. Negroes migrating from the deep South of the United States to the northern cities show an average increase in IQ of 4 points over four years. The rise is most marked in verbal tests and no change is observed in tests of ability to understand relations in space. This shows that verbal ability, presumably because it is an essential part of everyday life, is most easily acquired under these circumstances. A jump in IQ of from 9 to 12 points occurred in the Appalachian region of the United States between the 1920s and 1930s after the introduction of roads and schools. And the IQ of whites recruited to the U.S. Army rose by an average of 9 to 12 points between 1918 and 1943. The cultural differences between white America in 1918 and 1943 may be similar in degree to the cultural differences between negroes and whites in America today.

There is now evidence that Australian aborigines, often considered to be among the most "primitive" races of man, can be as intelligent as white Australians. The performance of aborigines and part-aborigines in IQ tests has been found by psychiatrist Barry Nurcombe of the University of New South Wales and psychologist Philip de Lacey of Wollongong University College to be determined by the amount of contact they have had with European culture rather than by their race.[5] Other studies have shown that the performance of aboriginal children adopted into white families does not differ from that of white children of similar social status. The reasons for the low performance of aborigines and part-aborigines in IQ tests is largely that the questions bear little relation to the normal modes of thinking of nomadic people.

President Johnson's Anti-Poverty Bill, made law in November, 1967, encouraged many attempts to help deprived children get ahead, and to raise their test scores. However, much of the work, which began on a wave of enthusiasm, was hastily and poorly planned. Many assumed that a crash course in the summer before school started would be sufficient to undo the effects of years of deprivation. Many of the programs had little education content and were designed in the naïve belief that free activity—the only thing many deprived children have plenty of—was an important need for these children. The majority of programs were modeled on upper-middle-class nursery methods that offer a broad experience but no training in depth. In a mere fifty hours of extra general teaching the deprived children were expected to catch up with their middle-class age group.

The few preschool groups for disadvantaged children that did produce any lasting results used a different method. They were based on the idea that if deprived children are to catch up at all they must be given more intense experiences of a kind that will equip them to go on learning by themselves. Poor ability with language severely slows down learning in deprived children. Any method to be effective must concentrate on improving ability with language so that children are not so easily left behind merely because they lack means of communicating with the world.

One of the most successful programs for improving the IQs of disadvantaged children has been organized by Rick Heber and colleagues at the University of Wisconsin, Madison. Heber was particularly interested in the children of mothers with low IQs. He found that the children of mothers with IQs below 80 gradually decline in IQ from 84 at the age of five to an average of about 66 at the age of fourteen. Heber selected forty mothers with IQs under 75 and divided them randomly into two groups of twenty. One group was offered an infant stimulation program and a maternal rehabilitation program. The teachers were people who lived nearby who were good with children, affectionate, and able to talk easily with the parents. The children began to attend a center at the age of three months, and each was given a teacher who stayed with the child until it was about fourteen months old. Then the child was gradually paired with other teachers and other children. Each teacher was responsible for the total care of the children but also had a prescribed schedule that included three main areas of teaching: math or problem-solving, talking, and reading. The teacher also had to maintain a rapport with the child's mother. The aim of the whole program was to prevent "those language, problem solving and achievement motivation deficits which are known to be common attributes of mild retardation.'' [6]

The mothers in the experimental group were also given a program to improve their homemaking and child-rearing skills. They were given help with reading, writing, and arithmetic and then job training in a large private nursing home. They learned laundry work, food service, and simple nursing. They also had group counseling sessions every day.

The results of this program of compensatory education began to be seen when the children reached the age of about twenty-two months, when the experimental group began to perform better in intelligence tests. The children in the experimental group had the extraordinarily high average IQ of 123 between the ages of two and four and a half as compared with an average IQ in the control group of 95. The children in the control group showed signs of dividing into two groups, one about normal (IQ of 100) and another with definitely subaverage performance. The large average gain in IQ of 27 points in the experimental group would probably be lost if these children were returned to the environment from which they were taken. But Heber is optimistic that they can be maintained as his program develops.

Other studies have shown that intervention on a smaller scale, in which staff spend about four hours a week with a child for two to three years and perhaps another hour a week with parents, can hold back the downward slide in IQ that occurs in children on the poverty line. This amount of time is less than 2.3 percent of the child's waking life between the age of birth and six years. This is a small part of the child's whole life experience and may be somewhere near the minimum for effective results.

The Coleman Report on Equality of Opportunity was published by the U.S. Department of Health, Education, and Welfare in 1966. Data had been collected from 654,000 pupils in four thousand schools in the United States. The report presented evidence suggesting that the differences in educational achievement and IQ of different social classes and racial groups were caused by biological differences as well as differences in social advantages. For example, American Indians were found on average to do consistently better in IQ tests than negroes. Yet according to Coleman's estimates the environment of the Indians was much worse than the environment of the negro. The conclusion drawn was that Indians are innately superior to negroes in IQ. Jensen says in his book *Genetics and Education* that his interest in heredity and IQ was strongly reinforced by reading the Coleman report. But a second report has been issued by the U.S. Department of Health, Education, and Welfare that takes the analysis of the data used by Coleman a stage further and shows that the original conclusions cannot be substantiated.

The second report, produced by George W. Mayeske and others, is called *A Study of Our Nation's Schools*. The report found, among many other detailed conclusions, that various social conditions could account for all the differences in school achievement between whites, negroes, Indians, Mexicans, Puerto Ricans, and Orientals in U.S. schools. Achievement was measured by tests of general knowledge, reading, math, and verbal and nonverbal ability. The report concluded: "No inferences can be made about the 'independent effect' of membership in a particular racial-ethnic group on academic achievement, for that membership, as it relates to academic achievement, is almost completely confounded with a variety of social conditions." [7]

A survey made in Britain by the Plowden committee came to a similar conclusion in recognizing the home circumstances as being most important in influencing the achievement of pupils. In 1967 the committee reported on education of children under twelve in Britain. It recommended more education for children and that more money be spent on schools in underprivileged areas.

The parental circumstances identified by the survey as being important were the literacy of the parents, the occupation of the father, and the number of children in the family. The child from a literate home enters school with an enormous advantage.

We are just beginning to understand the effects of upbringing on later intelligence. Gordon W. Miller of the University of London Institute of Education has shown that social class alone does not satisfactorily explain the differences in achievement of children. [8] But he has been able to identify some of the other important factors. He asked primary school children to fill in a questionnaire about themselves and correlated their answers with the results of school tests in verbal ability, English, and arithmetic.

Miller found two major factors that reduced the achievement of both boys and girls. Children who were submissive or who had dominant parents achieved less than others. Parents who spent little time with their children, did not give reasons for rules or punishments, and did not encourage reading or hobbies had a strong negative effect on their children's achievement. On the other hand, support from parents for staying on at school and for further education helped children achieve more. Confidence in ability to learn and tolerance of the children's arguments by parents were among other important factors correlated with achievement in both boys and girls.

Non-Europeans are generally found to do less well than Europeans on standard IQ tests. This led one South African psychologist to claim in 1939 that "the inferiority of the native in educability . . . limits considerably the proportion of natives who can benefit by education of the ordinary type beyond the rudimentary." [9] The work leading to this claim was subjected to devastating criticism by others who pointed out that no account was taken in the study of cultural background, schooling, or deficiencies of diet, which would certainly depress test scores.

This led to a search for a "culture-free" test. It was soon realized that a culture-free test was not possible, and so the mainstream testers settled for what has been called the "culture-fair" test. These tests use mainly abstract symbols in an effort to avoid the difficulty of using language. However, this approach has only succeeded in showing that there are other difficulties that cannot be evaded. For example, when one worker tried to apply a culture-fair test to Congolese he found that the results he obtained provided a good measure of their length of schooling but were much less well correlated with chronological age. Others have found it difficult, if not impossible, to use such tests with illiterates. In 1923 H. Gordon completed a classic study of English canal-boat children who had little formal schooling and were largely illiterate.[10] They showed average intelligence up to the age of six, but after that their IQs dropped as lack of schooling began to show an effect. This strong link between IQ and literacy suggests that IQ cannot be a measure of basic or innate intelligence but rather a function of school learning.

The development of the ability to read and write may be crucial in the development of intelligence and ability in abstract reasoning. Writing forces the mind to function at a more abstract level because, as one psychologist put it, "the spoken word stands for something, but the written word stands for something that stands for something."

Cultural differences of ability in IQ tests cannot necessarily be eliminated simply by using pictures of objects familiar to the cultural groups concerned. The whole idea of drawing on paper is outside the experience of many African tribespeople. They may fail to recognize a drawing of an object that is familiar to them as a carving in wood or ivory.

African mineworkers are often unable to grasp the significance of posters giving safety warnings specifically intended for them. When questioned about the message of a poster showing a hand with severed fingers, intended to warn of the danger of losing fingers caught in machinery, Africans replied "the poster teaches me how to write," "the man is counting with his fingers," "I should go and do likewise," and "I must wash my hands." [11] It is not difficult to imagine African mineworkers hurt in a mine accident being blamed for not understanding a warning using symbolism no one had bothered to explain to them. We take for granted skill in understanding symbols—from letters, digits, and signs of mathematics to the conventions of the comic strip—that we have learned in early childhood. There is nothing innate about these skills: they have to be learned.

Studies made in other cultures show that IQ tested in various ways can differ greatly from one culture to another. Psychologist W. Dennis has studied the ability of children between the ages of six and nine years of age to draw a man as part of a standard psychological test. The children were living in normal family environments in some fifty different cultures all over the world. The average IQs of these children, as measured by the draw-a-man test, varied from a high of 124 to a low of 52. Suburban children in America and England, children in a Japanese fishing village, and Hopi Indian children obtained the top average scores of 124. The low figure of 52 was obtained by children from a nomadic Bedouin tribe in Syria. A similar low average of 53 was scored by children of a nomadic Bedouin tribe in the Sudan. [12]

If no further thought were given to these figures it might be said that they demonstrated the innate genetic difference in measured intelligence between the races, showing that Arabs have inferior intelligence. The fact that Lebanese Arab children in Beirut scored an average IQ of 94 by the draw-a-man test might be taken as evidence to show that the more intelligent Arabs had migrated to the city.

This sort of argument, of course, completely overlooks the fact that the Muslim religion prohibits contact with graphic art. The children who did best in the draw-a-man test all came from cultures where children grow up in continuous contact with representational graphic art. City-living Arabs have a much greater contact with graphic Western art than other Arabs. Their different cultural experience almost certainly accounts for their better performance in these tests.

Cultural variation in intelligence can also be shown in other ways. Jean Piaget developed his theory of intelligence from observations of his own children and later extended them to other children living in Geneva. Piaget discovered a series of stages through which all children pass, from the first coordinated use of hand and eye to the understanding of logical relationships. A central idea in Piaget's scheme is that children reach a stage when they are ready to grasp the idea that quantities such as weight and volume are "conserved": that is to say, weight and volume remain the same despite a change in shape. For example, a pint of water is still a pint when it is transferred from a short glass to a long, thin glass. Understanding of the process of conservation is now recognized as a fundamental stage in the development of intelligence.

However, the actual age at which a child develops this kind of intelligence has been shown to vary with his environment. Psychologist D. Price-Williams was able to show this in a beautifully thought out study of pottery workers in Mexico. He predicted that the children of pottery workers would develop an understanding of conservation before other children of similar social background. The potters' children play with bits of clay from the age of five onward and three years later are trained in the preparation of clay for making pots. They have to prepare clay balls of a standard size, which are shaped to go into a mold. If the fit is not satisfactory, the clay has to be taken out, rolled into a ball once more, and reshaped. Price-Williams tested the abilities of the children of potters in two Mexican towns to understand conservation of number, liquid, weight, substance, and volume. In both towns the potters' children were better than other children at understanding the conservation of substance, and in one town they were also better at understanding all types of conservation.[13] This shows that with practice and training particular abilities can be acquired unusually early in life.

These experiments show that intelligence tests are complicated by the different experiences of perception gained by children in different cultures. These differences may even be acquired so early in life that the developing visual system of eye and brain is permanently affected. Cree Indians in Canada living the traditional life in tepees exist in an environment that does not contain many sharp horizontal or vertical lines, whereas Europeans in Canada, as elsewhere, live in a "carpentered" environment with many lines and angles. Tests of the perception of these two groups of people show that Euro-Canadians are less good at distinguishing oblique lines than Cree Indians, although the two groups are equally good at other tests of space perception.[14] The explanation of this curious observation may be that Cree Indians, because of the relative randomness of lines in their visual environments, have not developed a visual bias in favor of horizontals and verticals.

Another basic problem with intelligence testing is that the people being tested may not be accustomed to taking seriously arbitrary or abstract questions that may easily seem silly to someone with a pragmatic background. Africans from traditional cultures often cannot be made to feel competitive in IQ testing situations, so they may do badly because they do not feel any need to answer quickly. Even in the Hebridean Islands children answering intelligence tests in Gaelic are found to do it in a leisurely way with less feeling of competition than children from the city. Indeed, the IQ differences observed between city and country children, between Irish and English children, and between northern and southern negroes and between whites and blacks in the United States may be at least partly accounted for by such differences of attitude.

There is still a great deal of disagreement among psychologists and geneticists about the nature of IQ and the way it is inherited and acquired. I have simply tried to present in these chapters some of the evidence that throws doubt on the dogmatic hereditarian view that IQ is a stable measure that is 80 percent inherited. The more deeply the evidence is considered, the stronger these doubts appear to be. It is vital that these doubts should not be buried or forgotten. The practical and political consequences of educational policies based on the mistaken premise that intelligence is largely inherited could be vast and destructive.

CHAPTER 18

Your Status and Your Money

"If you're so smart, why aren't you rich?" is one way of asking what relationship there is, if any, between IQ and success. This cheeky question poses fundamental difficulties for those psychologists who stress the inheritance of IQ and its basic role in influencing the structure of society.

Professor Richard Herrnstein, author of *IQ in the Meritocracy,* stresses the connection between success and inherited ability. He spells out his argument like this:

1. If differences in mental abilities are inherited, and
2. If success requires those abilities, and
3. If earnings and prestige depend upon success,
4. Then social standing will be based to some extent on inherited differences between people.

Herrnstein foresees "a future in which social classes not only continue but become ever more solidly built on inborn differences." As society advances technologically, he believes that IQ will become even more important for success. "Even if every single job lost in automating a factory is replaced by a new job someplace else in a new technology, it is more than likely that some of those put out of the old jobs will not have the IQ for the new ones." Because of this, "in times to come, as technology advances, the tendency to be unemployed may run in the genes of a family about as certainly as bad teeth do now." [1]

The force of Herrnstein's argument depends upon the strength of his first two premises: that intelligence is inherited and that it is important to success in life. The first premise has already been shown to have important weaknesses. What about the second? In fact, the link between IQ and success is tenuous. Many people with high IQs are not rich and do not have prestigious jobs. And, more surprising, people with remarkably low IQs can achieve success even in academic study.

Many skills are needed in life outside school that just do not seem to be measured in any way by IQ tests. IQ tests also seem to be rather poor at predicting the ability of schoolchildren to win scholarships or obtain first-class degrees. Dr. Liam Hudson, professor of educational sciences at Edinburgh University in Scotland, found that the IQs of 24 percent of future scholarship winners were among the bottom 30 percent of pupils in one sample. IQ seemed to make no difference to a pupil's ability to win a scholarship. Tendency to work hard and breadth of interests outside the curriculum were the distinguishing features of future scholars.

Dr. Hudson found one boy who had an IQ lower than 80 percent of his classmates—some of whom left school without passing any of their school-leaving examinations—who gained an open scholarship to Cambridge University and went on to take a first-class degree in physics. His teachers had spotted his talents and predicted a brilliant career in physics, but the IQ tests showed no suspicion of this potential. Another boy followed by Hudson was only a little above average for his grade and his test results gave no hint of the brilliant future his teachers predicted. He won an open scholarship, took his degree in record time, and won the top mathematics prize at Cambridge. Hudson insists that these boys are not exceptions.[2]

American psychologist D. W. Mackinnon has suggested that when a person's IQ is above 115 to 125 it probably has little bearing on future intellectual achievement.[3] Psychologists in the United States are now looking for alternative means of predicting academic success. The most productive intellectuals have a capacity for obsessive work, focusing all their attention on one topic, whereas original thinkers may have less intellectual discipline than equally intelligent but less creative minds. When the abilities for unconventional thought and unrelenting application come together, then in theory we have a top productive thinker. But this is mostly supposition: tests have yet to be designed to identify these unusual minds.

A high IQ is of little help in getting a good, highly paid job. It does help, but so little that you can virtually forget it. The most superior fifth of the population in terms of IQ have incomes only 35 to 40 percent higher than the most inferior fifth, according to Jenck's calculations. This difference is very small when the best-paid fifth of Americans earn 600 percent more than the worst-paid fifth. And after allowances are made for family background and schooling, about half of this already small difference disappears.

If there is little benefit for the white person in having an above-average IQ, there is virtually none for the black man. It is much more difficult for the black middle-class father with a better-than-average IQ to pass any of his hard-won status on to his children, whatever their IQ. In the United States the son of a black middle-class man with above-average IQ usually ends up only a little better off than the average black man. Having the right parents with high IQ and good status does not seem to help blacks in the same way that it helps whites in the United States—perhaps to an employer blacks are more alike, whoever their fathers are. A white with the same IQ as a black will, on the whole, get a job with higher status.

Since the two basic premises of Herrnstein's thesis are open to such grave questions, there seems little point in worrying about his doom-laden predictions for the future of society. The real cause for worry is that the slim connection between IQ and success will be taken too seriously. If IQ tests were extensively used to select people for jobs, people with special talents not measured in IQ tests would be excluded. Then Herrnstein's predictions really might come true, but not quite in the way he thinks. The result would be a society rigidly divided into castes, with IQ tests serving as initiation ceremonies into the castes. The business of succeeding in the initiation ceremonies would become the primary objective and would guarantee other types of success. As a result, society would increasingly fossilize, while people became more and more obsessed with developing their IQ rather than with practical achievement. There is already a danger of this happening with college examinations, which may train people to pass examinations but do not necessarily help them to apply their knowledge in the broader context of society.

A person not only inherits a genetic endowment but may inherit property as well. While biologists have argued that intelligence, good health, and good nature are inherited through the genes, they have seldom stopped to consider how property is inherited. The possibility of a link between "good breeding" and an ample material inheritance is obvious enough, but there have been few proper investigations. Few economists have inquired into the economics of inheritance. And so the presumption that success in life is a consequence of inherited intelligence, rather than an ample financial inheritance, has gone largely unquestioned.

Theories of inherited civic worth and intellectual excellence propounded by biologists since Galton have, by exaggerating the importance of biological inheritance, covered up the important role that inheritance of property plays in maintaining social inequality. In effect, biological theories have been widely accepted as a rationalization of the social status quo. These biological theories may even have delayed the emergence of a full economic and social analysis of inheritance of money, land, and goods.

The endowment people inherit from their parents consists not only of property but also, for example, of their education and training, which may have been bought at extra expense. Social contacts are also an important part of a person's fortune, and school may provide many of these. If a father belongs to a trade union with restrictions on the entry of outsiders, then he may, in effect, endow his son with membership of the union. Similarly, children are able to make use of their parents' social and business connections to their advantage. The endowment parents are able to give their children will decide, broadly speaking, the income that the child is able to earn and the amount of property the child in turn is able to accumulate.

Another most important influence on the material and social endowment parents are able to give children is the number of other children in the family. In large families parents will have less time to spend with the children and less time to spend on helping them to get a good education and good jobs. The result is that children in large families have lower IQs.[4] Because of the extra drain on his resources, it is much more difficult for a man with a large family to accumulate property, and so he will also have less to leave his children.

The longer hours parents work, the less time they have to spend with their children and do what they can to aid their personal development, but the more money they have to endow their children with material advantages. Parents may go out to work hoping to earn more in order to give their children a better start, with the sad result that the children are neglected. This is particularly crucial in poor families, where the extra money gained simply helps to buy what to others are necessities.

Each man and woman brings into marriage a certain amount of property and a social endowment, which are seldom equal. The children benefit from the average of the endowments of their parents, which will be less than the larger of the two endowments—unless a major portion of the fortune is left to only one of the children, or there is an only child.

If men and women married at random, then children in the next generation would start off with an endowment that is nearer the average than that of their parents. This phenomenon, called regression to the mean (i.e., the average), also occurs when marriages are not completely random. However, the more like people marry like, the smaller the regression to the mean. Regression to the mean is a statistical phenomenon, although hereditarian biologists have sometimes made the grave error of arguing that regression to the mean is evidence for biological inheritance.

With each generation there will be some averaging of endowments, so that if no other forces were at work it might be expected that sooner or later everybody would be more or less equal in their fortunes. A large fortune amassed by good luck or through inherited good wits and hard work would be averaged away after a few generations. However we know that many modest fortunes, not to mention many greater fortunes, are maintained in families for generation after generation. There is no mystery about the way this is done. Two factors are important. First, men who have large fortunes tend to marry women who are also well endowed so that fortunes regress slowly, if at all, toward the mean by simple averaging. Second, laws and customs—such as the British practice of leaving the fortune to the eldest son (primogeniture)—influence the way in which fortunes change from generation to generation.

For the sake of argument, consider what would happen if family property had by law to be divided equally each generation between all the children, whether male or female. Property would then become much more equally divided between people in the population as a whole. In theory, if people married at random, after a few generations everybody would be endowed with an equal fortune. The speed of equalization would depend on the tendency of men and women with similar fortunes to marry each other. The only people with unusually large fortunes would be those people who by their ability or good luck were able to amass a fortune for themselves.

Now, suppose there were a law compelling people to leave all their property to their eldest child, whether the child was a daughter or a son. Properties would never be split between children but could be increased by marriage. They would go on growing bigger until all the property belonged to a very few people. And in theory, if the exercise could continue long enough without interruption by revolution or war, the property would all end up in the hands of one person. This would not happen if all property was always left to the eldest son (or in the absence of a son, the next male relative), because then two properties would never be joined together by marriage.

The situation in real life is a mixture of the two outlined above. The amount of concentration of wealth depends on the degree to which wealth is inherited without being divided between children and the degree to which wealthy men and women tend to marry each other (see more detailed analysis by Professor J. E. Meade).[5] In England (but not Scotland) and most states in the U.S.A. a person is free to dispose of his fortune virtually as he wishes. This freedom was obtained in England in 1688. In other European countries there are important restrictions on the way in which property can be disposed after death. In continental European countries the children and certain relatives of a person who has died are entitled to a reserved portion of the person's estate—the legitim—according to their degree of kinship and the claims of others. For example, if there are two children, each receives a third of the estate by right, and the remainder can be freely disposed. In England land can all be disposed of freely, but the custom of primogeniture is still common so that large estates tend to be preserved intact rather than split up. Entails may also be used under English law to tie up the property for the second generation of children. In France entails are illegal under the Napoleonic Code.

The number of children the rich and the poor choose to have is obviously another important factor affecting the distribution of wealth. If the rich chose to have larger families and chose to divide their fortune more equally between them, then there would be an increase in equality with each generation. But in most advanced countries in Europe and North America rich people tend to have small families, and this is an important factor in helping to preserve their wealth. An analysis of the achievements of British upper-class families supports the view that British society is dominated by a small elite caste.[6] An elite of about twenty-four thousand people out of some fifty-five million has for generations dominated the armed forces, the Church, the judiciary, the banks, and the civil and diplomatic services in Britain.

Although most of the available information about inheritance of property, assets and status concerns the wealthy and the elite, similar considerations apply to the middle classes. To take a simple example, the value of a person's house is dependent on the size of the deposit and mortgage he or she is able to pay. These in turn will be affected by the help parents are able to give in cash—some of which may be inherited—and in obtaining well-paying jobs for their children. How to work the system and get your son or daughter into a profession is obviously an invaluable asset that is passed down in professional families—just as a small shopkeeper may pass on assets, know-how and goodwill to his children.

Hereditarians argue that the poor are unhealthy, unintelligent, and often crazy or criminal, because they have inherited these weaknesses. If there is no sound scientific basis for these hereditarian arguments, as I have argued in this book, we must try to find a new and more convincing answer to the question: Why do poverty and deprivation continue in families for generation after generation? When the hereditarian assumptions are swept away, it is easy to see that poverty itself—a simple lack of cash and capital—is inherited. And with poverty goes environmental deprivation, the lack of opportunity to learn and grow as a person, which is just as surely passed on as one generation creates the home environment for the next.

We must now ask ourselves if the dice are not too heavily loaded against the poor and must ask what can be done to give poor children the *extra* opportunities needed to compensate for life in the ghetto and the slum. Society has a great deal to gain from improving the lives of the poor because problems of poverty, such as crime, spill over into society as a whole. What changes will best meet the problems of poor people and how welfare should be spent to improve the lives of the poor are a matter for political discussion and compromise.

MAN AND SUPERMAN

CHAPTER 19

Good Man, Bad Man, Madman, Superman: Who Do You Think YOU Are?

"Just before the doomed planet, Krypton, exploded to fragments, a scientist placed his infant son within an experimental rocket ship, launching it towards Earth." With these words Superman was born in *Action Comics* magazine in June, 1938. Throughout the Second World War and ever since, Superman has fought across the pages of *Action Comics* and the TV screens of America in defense of democracy. Superman was a symbol of courage and power that became part of the equipment of almost every American soldier.

Superman is a glorification of human power, intellectual and physical. Since Nietzsche first invented the idea, superman has been a symbol of man's superior potential. Belief in a kind of superman lies behind all scientific theories of intellectual superiority. *Genius* was Galton's chosen word for superman. The ideological drive behind the scientific theories of white superiority in IQ, such as those of Eysenck, Jensen, and Shockley, might reasonably be called a superman cult. The superman cult exaggerates man's innate potential and emphasizes instincts. It is racist, sexist, and elitist. Corollaries of the Superman cult are the cult of the bad man and the slave, the cult of the instinctive woman, the remorseless criminal, and the hereditary degenerate, and the belief that the underdog is innately predestined to his inferior existence and his unfortunate fate.

Superman in *Action Comics* is disguised as Clark Kent, the weakling bespectacled reporter. But as soon as there is a crisis Superman emerges with X-ray vision and the ability to leap over skyscrapers. It is a common psychological defense of superheroes to have a secret double identity. The reader may more easily identify with the superhero when the superhero also exists as an ordinary person. It is easy to develop similar fantasies about inheritance. Since few people know many details of their ancestry or anything significant about their heredity, they are at liberty to believe that they have inherited something rather special. And most people barely distinguish between their physical inheritance and the social position they have inherited. Such fantasies may be harmless in themselves, but they add up to a formidable social force. At best this force stabilizes society against disturbing changes, but it also fossilizes it.

These fantasies are most dangerous when they are bolstered by dubious biological and psychological theory and assembled into a superman cult. The apparently hard facts of biology easily provide the soft theories of society. The danger of these theories, such as the Y-chromosome theory of crime, the theory of inherited predisposition to smoking, lung cancer, and tuberculosis, and theories of inherited IQ or mental illness, lies in their spurious authority. Such authority is obtained by taking the facts and theories of one science and transposing them into another where they are not so easily questioned. Jacques Barzun, American academic and writer, has recognized this as the process by which racist theories gain their credibility. He writes in *Race: A Study of Superstition:*

> No system of race belief stays within its original limits. If it is a historical system, it drags in science and pseudo-science; if it is scientific it leans on historical or pseudo-historical facts; if philological, it relies on the other two disciplines. The proofs of any system are proofs only by assuming the truth of the other "facts", themselves assumed in a field beyond the one where the investigator originally bade you look.[1]

The elusive qualities of argument identified by Barzun are characteristic of hereditarian theories examined in this book. The basic device of these hereditarian theories is to use plausible genetic theory, including highly technical notions such as heritability quotients, to establish a case in some other discipline such as psychology or medicine.

In the absence of conclusive evidence, geneticists have typically been cautious in questioning plausible hereditary theories. They are understandably reluctant to disagree with the proposition that mental differences *may* exist between different races because there are no *theoretical* reasons either for or against the existence of such differences. People who are not familiar with genetics often feel that they have no alternative but to accept technical statements about human heredity because of the confident way these are made by scientists with the hereditarian approach. And so the hereditary theories of society develop by the accretion of inconclusive fact on plausible theory.

Hans Eysenck provides some outstanding examples of what might be called the Barzun phenomenon in his book *Race, Intelligence and Education.* In developing his hereditarian theory of IQ, Eysenck assumes that the genetic facts are established, conveniently dispensing with the necessity to consider fundamental objections to his theory. "The evidence," he said, "is well enough known to be mentioned only in passing." [2] He uses a similar approach in developing his theories of criminality and of smoking. However, the genetic evidence for all these theories has the property of appearing less and less substantial the more closely it is considered.

The Barzun phenomenon is also evident in the convenient historical assumptions Eysenck makes to support his theories of evolution of intelligence. Eysenck believes that American negroes are genetically inferior in IQ because their ancestors were too stupid to escape from slave traders, and that the most intelligent Irishmen left their country during the years of famine in the nineteenth century. These tidbits of historical supposition have little support from historians, and they are valueless as science because they are impossible to prove one way or the other. By such suppositions the cult of the superman, who escapes starvation and evades slave traders because of his innate intelligence, is built up.

In *Action Comics,* as in scientific theories, Superman has always defended the White Anglo-Saxon Protestant (Wasp) way of life. Superman fought for America in the Korean War and supported Senator McCarthy's anti-Communist crusade. Superman defends the political and social status quo.

In science the superman cult has done the same. Hereditarian science has rationalized the place of elites in society. This has prevented identification of the real causes of economic inequality and discussion of the issues that might be expected to stem from that. Public debate has been distorted by discussion of inheritance of IQ instead of social inequality, and by discussion of the inheritance of criminality instead of the cycle of deprivation that lies behind so much delinquency. And while the argument continues about genetic predispositions to smoking, cancer, and mental illness, the search for social remedies is delayed. Belief in inherited predestination encourages an unquestioning acceptance of society as it is, with so many rewards for the successful and so few for the unfortunate or the deprived. If this layer of spurious biological theory could be removed, it might be possible to debate whether society could be changed to give the underdog a better chance. When political biology is put aside, the real politics can begin.

The dreadful irony of the hereditarian view of society is that if enough people believe in it they might make it come true, regardless of scientific discrepancies in the arguments that lie behind it. Only continued public discussion of the question can avoid such a takeover bid by superman. If educational and social policies are based on the theory that a large section of the population is innately inferior in intelligence—or that it is different in any way—then the logical solution is to give that section of the population special and separate facilities suited to its apparent needs. The danger is that such separate facilities, despite good intentions, would be inferior. This does not mean that disadvantaged sections of the population do not need special education facilities, but they need special extra facilities that recognize their potential as well as their humanity and dignity. And these facilities must not be based on an assumption of inferiority. To be effective, such extra facilities would probably have to be available from the first or second year of life and continued until teen age.

Superman of Krypton and *Action Comics* was born with astounding powers. As a toddler he astonished doctors by lifting chests of drawers above his head, and as a youth he could vault skyscrapers and run faster than an express train. These are impossible feats. To create a Superman such as Clark Kent is obviously impossible. Nevertheless, scientific principles might perhaps be used to develop a lesser breed of supermen.

Hereditarians who fear "genetic decay" argue that if only we could create a superior race of men—or at least discourage breeding of inferior human types—the future of the human race would be assured. Let us assume for a moment that our aim is to create a superior type of person and that all the facilities of science are at our disposal. How might a scientist in the year 2000 set about this task?

A genetic engineer would select from among existing people the best physical and intellectual specimen he could find to be a genetic donor. As a scientist, he might choose someone with the brain of Einstein or Bertrand Russell, if such could be found, although this is not everyone's idea of a superman. Others might consider that a top footballer or world champion boxer such as Muhammad Ali might be the best genetic donor. Or if hoping to create a superwoman, our genetic engineer would be faced with the problem of whether to select a Marie Curie or a Marilyn Monroe.

Assuming that a suitable donor could be found, the genetic engineer of the future would take a single cell, perhaps from the blood, or perhaps from the intestine, of the donor. The problem then is to remove the nucleus of the cell, which carries the genetic instructions, and inject it into a fresh human egg cell from which the nucleus has been removed. Dr. J. B. Gurdon of Oxford University has done this operation successfully in frogs many times, and the eggs have developed into normal adult frogs. But the process, called cloning, has not yet been attempted in people because, apart from any ethical objections, the human egg is too small. In the frog the operation is done using microsurgical apparatus, but it is doubtful if this could be scaled down sufficiently to do the same operation on the human egg.

However, the time can be foreseen when molecular biologists may be able to use the human sperm to carry a donor nucleus into the egg. Eventually it may be possible to dismantle the human sperm chemically and reassemble it again with the nucleus of an adult cell wrapped up inside. These artificial sperm could then be used to fertilize eggs whose own nuclei had been knocked out by ultraviolet irradiation. This human egg would, accidents apart, be an exact replica of the human egg from which the donor person originally developed.

The egg would then be placed in the womb of a foster mother carefully chosen for her good health. The foster mother's own heredity would have no influence on the outcome, provided she was healthy and there were no blood-group problems. A caesarean birth would probably be preferred to avoid the possibility of accidental damage during delivery. If all went well, a perfect baby would be born. What would the genetic engineer do then? His special expertise is exhausted and he must find some parents for the child.

Assuming he managed to do that, would the child inevitably develop the scientific genius of Einstein, Russell, or Marie Curie—or the brilliant talent of Marilyn Monroe or Muhammad Ali? If this experiment could be done, it would answer the basic question of how important heredity is in deciding human intelligence and character. Professor J. B. S. Haldane, a brilliant biologist but a dedicated hereditarian, considered that cloning could "raise the possibilities of human achievement dramatically." He believed most clones would be made from people over fifty when their achievements in life could be assessed, except for athletes and dancers who might be cloned when they were younger. Haldane considered that clones would be made from people who have excelled in socially acceptable accomplishments. He also thought it might be of value to clone particular kinds of people, for example those who lack a sense of pain or people who, like Eastern yogis, can control their unconscious bodily functions. Cloning has also been taken seriously by Lord Rothschild, a distinguished biologist turned industrialist who was at one time at the head of former British Prime Minister Edward Heath's government think tank. He has foreseen the creation of a Commission for Genetical Control to get applications from those who want to clone themselves.

Enthusiasm for cloning is based on the assumption that intelligence and talent are largely inherited with the genes—it is based on the old "hard machine" concept of human heredity. However, it seems most unlikely to me that it would ever be possible to reproduce a person by cloning with any accuracy—least of all people with exceptional talent who probably develop from a fortuitous combination of hereditary potential combined with an unusual environment. Each of us is unique not just because we inherit a unique combination of genes but because we are born into a special environment that can never be repeated exactly at a later time. The idea that cloning is feasible is based on hereditarian ideas—indeed, it is the ultimate hereditarian fantasy. The most that cloning could hope to do is to provide the raw material that might make an Einstein or a Muhammad Ali if the right environmental conditions could be found. But I would hazard the guess that if a molecular biologist were to clone a thousand Einsteins or Muhammad Alis and place them in families chosen at random, not one of them would excel like the stock they came from and the majority would be quite ordinary people.

At first sight there may seem to be nothing unethical in attempting cloning if it were done with the full knowledge and consent of a couple who intended to bring up the child themselves. But such technical manipulations would always carry an extra risk of something going wrong that might damage the egg and so the baby. Such extra risks could not compensate for any gain in being able to choose a child with particular physical characteristics. And there is another sort of objection. Would children who were cloned be able to live with the expectations their parents had of them? Assuming that the parents knew the type of stock they had selected—and the exercise would be pointless otherwise—they would expect the child to develop into a brilliant musician, physicist, athlete, or whatever. This could expose the child to quite intolerable pressures to succeed that might threaten the child's sanity, however "sane" the biological stock from which the child was derived.

Another scientific approach to the development of superman that need not await technical developments is selective breeding. The methods of the animal breeder might be applied to man. In theory this might even be done without too gross interference with human liberty by simply persuading married couples to use sperm taken from "superior" men. Healthy, sane men with high IQs would presumably be chosen as breeding material. H. J. Muller, U.S. geneticist who won the Nobel Prize in 1947 for his work on the artificial production of mutations, suggested that the sperm of genetically superior males be used for artificial insemination. In this way the race might be improved, he thought. Muller wrote: "There is no physical, legal or moral reason why the sources of the germ cells used should not represent the germinal capital of the most truly outstanding and eminently worthy persons known." [3] Muller stressed that the program should be operated only by "voluntary choice." However, Muller himself inadvertently illustrates one of the difficulties facing such a program. In what way would superior men be selected to donate their sperm? In Muller's first book on the subject, published in 1935, he included in his list of suitable men Lenin, Marx, and Sun Yat-sen. In a later book, published in 1959 after Muller was disillusioned with Russia, these three names were dropped and Einstein and Lincoln added. [4]

Muller's change of mind illustrates the problems facing people who are seriously considering selective breeding. First of all, they must decide whether they want their child to be a Lenin or a Lincoln, a football player or a musician. Then they and the child must live with the decision for the rest of their lives. If such selective breeding were really to work and make any difference to the next generation, then the danger is that it would be packed with yesterday's men—out of fashion and unsuited to the problems of the day. But of course this whole idea is absurd. It takes much more than the right combination of genes to create a Lenin or a Lincoln. In any case, most couples would certainly prefer to bring their own children into the world. The last thing many people would want in their family—even if it were possible—is a budding Einstein or a Marilyn Monroe.

If a voluntary breeding scheme did not work, there is the danger that one of the schemes suggested by Shockley as a thinking exercise might be considered—perhaps his child-rationing scheme based on the deci-child certificate. But to enforce such a plan would require a police state with unprecedented powers to intervene in private life. It can scarcely be worth risking our democratic freedoms in order to try out a hypothetical scheme for increasing national intelligence and talent. Such breeding schemes are science fiction fantasies that overlook the social facts of life. People live and reproduce in families, and they do not want to be treated like breeding stock.

Eugenic programs aimed at reducing the numbers of "inferior" people by sterilization are easier to implement than positive breeding programs, and such a program has been implemented recently in the United States under the guise of population control. Following an inquiry in the U.S. District Court in Washington in June, 1974, Judge Gerhardt A. Gesell said, "There is uncontroverted evidence in the record that minors and other incompetents have been sterilized with federal funds and that an indefinite number of poor people have been improperly coerced into accepting a sterilization operation under threat that various federally supported welfare benefits would be withdrawn unless they submitted to irreversible sterilization." [5] Judge Gesell found that some 100,000 to 150,000 poor people were sterilized in 1972 with federal welfare support channeled through the Department of Health, Education, and Welfare (HEW) and the Office for Economic Opportunity (OEO). These programs were intended to be voluntary, but many poor people, teen-agers, and mentally retarded people did not know what was being done to them. The sterilization program was revealed following a legal action by two illiterate sisters from Alabama, aged twelve and fourteen, who were sterilized without their knowledge in June, 1973. Judge Gesell ruled that minors and incompetents cannot fully understand the detrimental effects of sterilization. So sterilization must always be involuntary for them and therefore illegal. *The New England Journal of Medicine* (July 4, 1974) welcomed the judgment and commented: "Too many medical programs of sterilization have been used in a coercive manner to achieve highly questionable goals of population control among poor people on welfare." [6] It is, of course, intolerable in a free society that people should be coerced into being sterilized. It is a tribute to the U.S. National Welfare Rights Organization and the U.S. legal system that this abuse has been rapidly stopped.* The doctors who performed these sterilizations have been seriously misled by the hereditarian view of society prevailing in science. But HEW and OEO also carry a grave

---

* The relevant cases were heard in the U.S. District Court, Washington, D.C., in June, 1974. They are: *Relf* vs. *Weinberger*, Civil Action No. 73-1557; *National Welfare Rights Organization* vs. *Weinberger*, Civil Action No. 74-243).

responsibility because they failed to issue ethical guidelines for sterilization.[7]

Another quite different suggestion for dealing with the problem of poor people with subnormal intelligence has been made by Eysenck. He suggests that children with low IQs be given drugs such as glutamic acid to strengthen their nervous system and so increase their intelligence. The suggestion has a rational hypothetical basis in that glutamic acid plays an important part in the chemistry of the brain. It is necessary for the synthesis of acetylcholine, a substance essential for the production of electrical changes when messages pass along the nerves. Several claims have been made that glutamic acid will improve the IQ of both retarded and normal children. However, the majority of scientific investigations into this claim have been of a rather poor quality. As many investigations have found no benefit from glutamic acid as have found benefit. Many of the investigations employed no control group of subjects who were not given the glutamic acid, and so a valid comparison is difficult to make. Others were not double-blind—that is, the investigator knew which subjects were being given the active drug and so could be unconsciously biased in his assessments of the effect of the drug. But even if glutamic acid does help some children gain in IQ—which is a matter of serious doubt— the gains cannot be made without formal teaching being given at the same time. Glutamic acid *might* assist the development of IQ, but it will never replace the teacher. And the same conclusion is likely to apply to any other drug that may be found to influence the function of the brain favorably. There will never be a wonder drug for developing IQ—the concept is absurd.

There is also the possibility of undesirable side effects from drugs used to increase intelligence. These will need to be most carefully examined before any drug is ever used on a wide scale for this purpose. Sodium glutamate, which is virtually identical to glutamic acid, has been identified as the cause of Chinese restaurant syndrome. This is a painful cramp in the back of the neck commonly experienced by people after they have drunk wonton soup or eaten other Chinese dishes containing large quantities of sodium glutamate as a flavoring. Sodium glutamate has also been shown to damage the growing brains of rats and monkeys [8] and so has been removed from baby food in many countries of the world. Nevertheless, Eysenck is enthusiastic. He "envisages a world" in which all children with "low IQs" (he specifies 100 or less) are given the drug.

All these superscientific approaches to the creation of a superrace or a supersociety have some awkward catch. They are shortcuts to nowhere. Is there some more practical, more realistic way that might be used to improve "human quality"? Yes, there is. It can be done with humanity through relationships between people.

Psychologists such as Rick Heber who have persisted in their research into preschool education, despite the failure of the Headstart program, are now getting results. These show that poor children can be helped to develop if together with their mothers they are given a regular program of play activities. It is vital for the success of these programs that the mother is included so that she can carry the program over into the home. This is just the beginning of what could become a new social engineering that helps mothers—if they want help—to bring out the best in their children. A national program should be possible when further research has discovered the best method of teaching constructive play. Such methods will tap great hidden reserves of ability in our society and enable many more children to benefit from school education.

Enormous improvements have been made in the health of people in all Western nations through the increased understanding and control of the environmental causes of disease. Public health measures controlled the tuberculosis that plagued our cities long before drugs became available to treat the disease. As a result of these environmental improvements, no one is interested anymore in whether a predisposition to tuberculosis is inherited—we know that public health measures control the infection. These public health measures became possible when administrators and politicians understood that this type of disease was caused by infection in the environment and not by inherited human weakness.

A similar connection exists between the human mind and the environment it is exposed to. We are groping toward a scientific understanding of the effect of people on each other in the home and in society. We are just beginning to understand how intelligent, sane, and healthy people develop. Eventually it will be possible to exploit this knowledge systematically and so improve "human quality" and the quality of life for many people. We must also continue to search for the causes of crime, alcoholism, and drug addiction in the social environment. If these are environmental problems—and I believe they are—then there are environmental solutions.

For too long we have been told by lords of the manor, politicians, and scientific supermen what they think we should be. We have been told who is fit to govern and who is fit to breed. These men have fostered the view that humanity is a hard machine programmed to develop according to a predetermined genetic code. We often unconsciously accept this view of ourselves and our children without realizing how weak its scientific basis is. But we are not slaves of our biological inheritance. We can change our environment and eventually our lives.

Who do you think you are? Who do you want to be?

Notes

Introduction

1. Theodore Roszak, *The Making of a Counter Culture* (New York: Doubleday, 1969; London, Faber and Faber, 1970).

Chapter 2

1. Zhores A. Medvedev, *The Rise and Fall of T. D. Lysenko* (New York and London: Columbia University Press, 1969).
2. Friedrich Nietzsche, *Thus Spake Zarathustra,* translated by R. J. Hollingdale (London and Baltimore: Penguin, 1961).
3. Walter Kaufmann, *Nietzsche: Philosopher, Psychologist, Antichrist* (New York: Random House, Vintage Books, 1968).
4. Ernst Haeckel, *The Wonders of Life* (New York: Harper, 1904), pp. 118–119.
5. Dr. Wilhelm Frick, quoted by Dunn (below) from *Archiv für Rassen-und-Gesellschaftsbiologie* 27: 451.
6. L. C. Dunn, "Cross Currents in the History of Human Genetics," *American Journal of Human Genetics* 14 (1962): 1–13.
7. Otto von Verschuer, letter to *American Journal of Human Genetics* 14 (1962): 309–310.
8. Eliot Slater, "German Eugenics in Practice," *Eugenics Review* 27 (1936): 289–295.
9. Dr. Erwin Baur, Dr. Eugen Fischer, and Dr. Fritz Lenz, *Human Heredity* (London: George Allen & Unwin Ltd., and New York: Macmillan, 1931). German edition (Munich: I. F. Lehmanns Verlag, 1927).
10. Francis Galton, *Inquiries into Human Faculty and Its Development,* 3rd ed. (London: J. M. Dent & Sons, Ltd. 1908).
11. Francis Galton, "Eugenics, Its Definition, Scope and Aims," *Sociological Papers* (London, 1905). Also published in *Essays in Eugenics* (The Eugenics Society, 1909).

12. Francis Galton, *Memories of My Life* (London: Methuen & Co., 1908).

13. Francis Galton, *Hereditary Genius* (London: Macmillan & Co., 1869).

14. Ibid.

15. Francis Galton, "Hereditary Improvement," *Frazer's Magazine* VII (January, 1873): 116–130.

16. Francis Galton, *The Eugenic College of Kantsaywhere* (1910). Galton destroyed the manuscript of *Kantsaywhere* when it was turned down by a publisher. But extensive fragments have been preserved and published in Karl Pearson's *Life, Letters and Labours of Francis Galton* IIIA (1930), pp. 411–425. Another useful biography of Galton is also to be found in C. P. Blacker's *Eugenics: Galton and After* (London: Gerald Duckworth and Co., 1952).

17. L. S. Penrose, Presidential address, "The Influence of the English Tradition in Human Genetics," *Proceedings of the Third International Congress of Genetics* (Baltimore: Johns Hopkins Press, 1966).

18. Harry H. Laughlin, "A Statement of the Basic Problem, and of the Main Findings in the Analysis of Pan-American Immigration Control and Policy" (Washington, D. C.: Eugenics Record Office of the Carnegie Institute of Washington, 1936); and Oscar Handlin, *Race and Nationality in American Life*, pp. 97–98, 131–133, 137–138.

19. Charles B. Davenport, "The Effects of Race Intermingling," *Proceedings of the American Philosophical Society* LVI (April 13, 1917): 367.

20. Ibid.

21. Paul Popenoe and Roswell H. Johnson, *Applied Eugenics* (New York: Macmillan, 1923).

22. Charles B. Davenport and M. Steggerda, "Race Crossing in Jamaica" (Washington, D. C.: Carnegie Institute of Washington, *Publication # 395*, 1929).

23. H. L. Shapiro, "Descendants of the Mutineers of the Bounty," Memoirs of the Bernice P. Bishop Museum, Honolulu, vol. 11, no. 1 (1929).

24. L. C. Dunn and A. M. Tozzer, Papers of the Peabody Museum of American Archaeology and Ethology, vol. 11 (Cambridge, Mass.: Harvard University, 1928): 90.

25. M. J. Herskovits, *The American Negro: A Study in Racial Crossing* (New York: Knopf, 1928).

26. C. D. Darlington, *Genetics and Man* (London: first published by George Allen & Unwin Ltd., 1964; revised for Penguin Books, 1966, and currently available); New York, Macmillan, 1964; Schocken Books, 1969.

27. Dr. Erwin Baur, et al., *Human Heredity*.

28. UNESCO statement published in *The Race Concept* (Paris: UNESCO, 1951).

29. Ibid.

30. William B. Provine, "Geneticists and the Biology of Race Crossing," *Science*, vol. 182 (1974): 790–796.

31. Ibid.

32. Konrad Lorenz, *Civilised Man's Eight Deadly Sins* (London: Methuen and Co., 1973).

Chapter 3

1. R. J. Herrnstein, *IQ in the Meritocracy* (Boston and Toronto: Little Brown and Co.; London: Allen Lane, 1973).
2. C. D. Darlington, *The Evolution of Man and Society* (New York: Simon and Schuster, 1969; London: George Allen & Unwin Ltd., 1969).
3. C. D. Darlington, *The Facts of Life* (London: George Allen & Unwin Ltd., 1953; New York: Schocken Books, 1969).
4. Ibid.
5. John B. Watson, *Behaviorism* (New York: Norton, 1924).
6. J. McVicker Hunt, ed., *The Role of Experience in Human Intelligence* (New Brunswick, N. J.: Transaction Inc., 1972).
7. Arthur R. Jensen, "How Much Can We Boost IQ and Scholastic Achievement?" *Harvard Educational Review,* vol. 39, no. 1 (February, 1969).
8. Herrnstein, *IQ in the Meritocracy.*
9. Ibid.
10. William Shockley, "Human Quality Problems and Research Taboos." Text of address to the National Academy of Sciences (Washington, D. C.) given in the spring of 1968. Text supplied by Dr. Shockley to author and dated February 26, 1969.
11. Ibid.
12. H. J. Eysenck, *Race, Intelligence and Education* (London: Maurice Temple Smith, 1971; New York, Library Press, 1971).
13. Ibid., p. 148.
14. Darlington, *The Facts of Life,* p. 289.
15. Kate Millett, *Sexual Politics* (New York: Avon, 1971; London: MacGibbon and Kee Ltd., 1972), p. 222.
16. John Stuart Mill, "Principles of Politics and Economics."
17. J. Arthur Thomson, *Heredity* (London: John Murray, 1908).
18. Sir Cyril Burt, "The Genetic Determination of Differences in Intelligence: A Study of Monozygotic Twins Reared Together and Apart," *British Journal of Psychology,* vol. 57 (1966): 137–153.

Chapter 4

1. Alfred Jost, "Development of Sexual Differences," *Science Journal,* June, 1970.
2. Gabriel Khorobkhov, quoted by James Coote in "When Is a Woman Not a Woman," *The Sunday Telegraph* (London: September 4, 1966): 11.
3. John Money and Anke A. Ehrhardt, *Man and Woman, Boy and Girl* (Baltimore and London: Johns Hopkins University Press, 1972).

Chapter 5

1. Mr. Justice Ormrod, quoted in *The Times* Law Report February 3, 1970 (London: *The Times,* published by Times Newspapers Ltd.).

2. Ibid.
3. Ibid.
4. *The Lancet,* editorial, "Sex, Intersex and the Law," vol. 1 (London: January 17, 1970): 128.
5. Martin Roth and J. R. B. Ball, "Psychiatric Aspects of Intersexuality," in *Intersexuality in Vertebrates Including Man,* C. N. Armstrong and A. J. Marshall, eds. (London and New York: Academic Press, 1964).
6. John Money and Anke A. Ehrhardt, *Man and Woman, Boy and Girl.*
7. Ibid.
8. Harry Benjamin, "Clinical Aspects of Transsexualism in the Male and Female," *American Journal of Psychotherapy,* vol. 18 (1964): 458–469.
9. Roth and Ball, "Psychiatric Aspects of Intersexuality."
10. Virginia Prince, from my own notes of the Gender Identity Conference held in London, England, July, 1969, sponsored by the Erikson Educational Foundation of New York and the Albany Trust of London.
11. Ingebord L. Ward, "Prenatal Stress Feminises and Demasculinises the Behaviour of Males," *Science,* vol. 175: 82–84.
12. John B. Calhoun, "Death Squared: The Explosive Growth and Demise of a Mouse Population," *Proceedings of the Royal Society of Medicine,* vol. 66 (London: January, 1973): 80.

Chapter 6

1. A. C. Kinsey, W. B. Pomeroy, C. E. Martin, and P. H. Gebhard, *Sexual Behavior in the Human Male* (Philadelphia: W. B. Saunders Co., 1948).
2. H. J. Eysenck, *Crime and Personality* (London: Paladin Books, Granada Publishing, 1970; first published London: Routledge and Kegan Paul Ltd., 1964).
3. C. D. Darlington, *Genetics and Man.*
4. André Gide, *If It Die (Si le grain ne meurt;* first published Penguin edition, 1920).
5. Quoted by Roth and Ball, "Psychiatric Aspects of Intersexuality," from André Maurois, *A la Recherche de Marcel Proust* (Paris: Hachette, 1949).
6. Irving Bieber, *Homosexuality: A Psychoanalytic Study of Male Homosexuals* (New York: Basic Books, 1967).
7. Eva Bene, "On the Genesis of Male Homosexuality," *British Journal of Psychiatry,* vol. 111 (1965): 803–813.
8. A. C. Kinsey, W. B. Pomeroy, C. E. Martin, and P. H. Gebhard, *Sexual Behavior in the Human Female* (Philadelphia: W. B. Saunders Co., 1953).
9. F. E. Kenyon, *British Journal of Psychiatry,* vol. 114 (1968): 1337.
10. Eva Bene, "On the Genesis of Female Homosexuality."
11. Malvina W. Kremer and Alfred Rifkin, work described in "Research with Adolescents Sheds New Light on Early Lesbianism," *Science News,* vol. 96 (July 19, 1969): 45.
12. Dr. Irwin Bernstein, work described in "Status Seeking Hormones," *Newsweek* (August 23, 1973): 46.

13. F. J. Kallman, "Comparative Twin Study of the Genetic Aspects of Male Homosexuality," *Journal of Nervous and Mental Disease,* vol. 115 (1952): 282–298. F. J. Kallman, "Twin Sibships and the Study of Male Homosexuality," *American Journal of Human Genetics,* vol. 4 (1952): 136–146.

14. D. J. West, *Homosexuality* (London: Penguin, 1971).

Chapter 7

1. H. A. Moss, "Sex, Age and State as Determinants of Mother-Infant Interaction," in K. Danziger, ed., *Readings in Child Socialisation* (London: Pergamon Press, 1970).

2. A. W. H. Buffery and J. A. Grey, "Sex Differences in the Development of Perceptual and Linguistic Skills," in C. Ounsted and D. C. Taylor, eds., *Gender Differences: Their Ontogeny and Significance* (Edinburgh: Churchill, 1967).

3. E. E. Maccoby, ed., "Sex Differences in Intellectual Functioning," in *The Development of Sex Differences* (London: Tavistock Publications, 1967).

4. David M. Levy, *Maternal Overprotection* (New York: Columbia University Press, 1943).

5. Ann Oakley, *Sex, Gender and Society* (London: Maurice Temple Smith, 1972).

6. Matina Horner et al., "Femininity and Successful Achievement: A Basic Inconsistency," chap. 3 in *Feminine Personality and Conflict* (Belmont, Calif.: Brooks/Cole, 1970). Also published in *Roles Women Play: Readings Towards Women's Liberation,* M. Grasskoff, ed. (Belmont, Calif.: Brooks/Cole, 1971).

7. Helen Hacker, "Women as a Minority Group," *Social Forces* (Chapel Hill: University of North Carolina Press, 1951), pp. 60–69.

8. Dr. L. Thimm, "Leistungsprinzip oder Neider mit den Frauen," *Die Ärtztin,* vol. 10, no. 1 (January, 1934), pp. 3–4 and 28.

9. Adolf Hitler, quoted in *N. S. Frauenbuch (Nazi Women's Handbook)* (München: J. F. Lehmanns, 1934), pp. 10–11.

10. Dr. Erwin Baur, et al. *Human Heredity.*

11. Ibid.

12. C. D. Darlington, *Genetics and Man.*

13. Ibid.

14. Ibid.

15. Kate Millett, *Sexual Politics,* p. 221.

Chapter 8

1. Cesare Lombroso, *Introduction to Gina Lombroso Ferrara: Criminal Man According to the Classification of Cesare Lombroso* (New York: Putnam, 1911).

2. Charles Darwin, *The Descent of Man* (London: John Murray, 1871), p. 137.

3. Charles Goring, *The English Convict* (London: Her Majesty's Stationery Office, 1913).

4. Ernest Hooton, *The American Criminal: An Anthropological Study* (Cambridge, Mass.: Harvard University Press, 1939).

5. F. W. Masters and D. C. Greaves, work described by Christine Doyle in "Does the Face Make the Criminal," *The Observer* (London: June 18, 1967).

6. H. J. Eysenck, *Crime and Personality*, p. 142.

7. Professor William Shockley, letter to members of the National Academy of Sciences (Washington, D. C.) dated April 23, 1969, signed by Walter C. Alvarez, John H. Northrup, John B. deC. M. Saunders, W. Shockley, and with reservations by Sheldon Glueck.

8. R. L. Dugdale, *The Jukes,* 4th ed. (G. P. Putnam, 1888).

9. Henry H. Goddard, *The Kallikak Family* (Macmillan, 1912; reprinted 1939). Henry H. Goddard, "In Defense of the Kallikak Study," *Science* (June 5, 1942).

10. Leon Radzinowicz, *History of the English Criminal Law,* 3 vols. (London: Stevens, 1948–1956).

11. Clifford Shaw and H. McKay, *Juvenile Delinquency and Urban Areas* (Chicago: University of Chicago Press, 1942).

Chapter 9

1. Francis Wyndham, *The Sunday Times* (London: Times Publications Ltd., October 19, 1969).

2. Professor Dr. J. Lange, *Crime As Destiny: A Study of Criminal Twins.* Foreward by J. B. S. Haldane (London: George Allen & Unwin Ltd., 1931); original German edition (Leipzig: Georg Thieme Verlag, 1929).

3. Ibid.

4. H. J. Eysenck, *Crime and Personality,* chap. 3.

5. J. B. S. Haldane, Foreward to *Crime As Destiny.*

6. Karl O. Christiansen, "Mobility and Crime among Twins," *International Journal of Criminology and Penology,* vol. 1 (1973): 31–45.

Chapter 10

1. Mary Wollstonecraft Shelley, *Frankenstein* (London: Dent and Sons, 1921; first published 1818).

2. Albert Wilson, *The Child of Circumstance* (London: John Bale, Sons and Danielsson, 1929).

3. Ibid.

4. M. D. Casey, C. E. Blank, D. R. K. Street, L. J. Segall, J. H. McDougall, P. J. McGrath, and J. L. Skinner, "YY Chromosomes and Anti-social Behaviour," *The Lancet,* vol. 2 (1966): 859.

5. Patricia A. Jacobs, W. H. Price, and W. M. Court Brown, "Chromosome Studies on Men in Maximum Security Hospital," *Annals of Human Genetics,* vol. 31 (London: 1968): 344.

6. W. H. Price and P. B. Whatmore, "Behaviour Disorders and Patterns of Crime among XYY Males Identified at a Maximum Security Hospital," *British Medical Journal,* vol. 1 (1967): 533.

7. *London Evening News* (August 30, 1967).

8. "Studies on the Human Y Chromosome," *Medical Research Council Annual Report* (April, 1966—March, 1967), p. 41. (London: Her Majesty's Stationery Office).

9. M. D. Casey, L. J. Segall, D. R. K. Street, and C. E. Blank, "Sex Chromosome Abnormalities in Two State Hospitals for Patients Requiring Special Security," *Nature,* vol. 209 (London: 1966): 641.

10. M. D. Casey, D. R. K. Street, L. J. Segall, and C. E. Blank, "Patients with Sex Chromosome Abnormalities in Two State Hospitals," *Annals of Human Genetics,* vol. 32 (1968): 53.

11. W. M. Court Brown, W. H. Price, and P. A. Jacobs, "The XYY Male," *British Medical Journal,* vol. 4 (1968): 513.

12. E. P. Bellamy, "Unanswered Questions in Human Criminal Behavior Patterns," *The Times* (London: January 5, 1972).

13. "Patients' Rights: Harvard Is Site of Battle over X and Y Chromosomes," *Science* (November 22, 1974): 715; "Controversy over XYY Screening," *Medical Tribune* (January 15, 1975): 1; "XXY–XYY Syndromes: Gauging the Odds," *Medical World News* (September 6, 1974).

14. Johannes Nielsen, "Prevalence and a Two and a Half Years Incidence of Chromosome Abnormalities among All Males in a Forensic Psychiatric Clinic," *British Journal of Psychiatry,* vol. 119 (1971): 503–512.

15. J. Kahn, W. I. Carter, N. Dernley, and E. T. O. Slater, "Chromosome Studies in Remand Home and Prison Populations," in *Criminological Implications of Chromosome Abnormalities.* D. J. West, ed. (Cambridge, England: Institute of Criminology, 1969).

Health: Introduction

1. Elsie M. Widdowson, "Mental Contentment and Physical Growth," *The Lancet,* vol. 1 (London: June 16, 1951): 1316.

2. Lytt I. Gardner, "Deprivation Dwarfism," *Scientific American* (1973).

Chapter 11

1. H. J. Eysenck, *Smoking, Health and Personality* (London: Weidenfeld and Nicolson, 1965).

2. R. Doll and A. B. Hill, "Mortality in Relation to Smoking: Ten Years' Observations on British Doctors," *British Medical Journal* (May 30, 1964): 1399; (June 6, 1964): 1460.

3. James Shields, *Monozygotic Twins* (London: Oxford University Press, 1962).

4. H. J. Eysenck, *Race, Intelligence and Education,* p. 81.

5. Rune Cederlof et al., *Archives of Environmental Health* (Chicago, 1966 and 1967).

6. The Royal College of Physicians, *Smoking and Health Now* (London: Pitman Medical and Scientific Publishing Co. Ltd., 1971).

7. Anne Roe, "The Adult Adjustment of Children of Alcoholic Parents Raised in Foster Homes," *The Quarterly Journal of Alcohol Studies*, vol. 5 (1944): 378–393.

8. D. W. Goodwin, F. Schulsinger, L. Hermansen, S. B. Guze, and G. Winokur, "Alcohol Problems in Adoptees Raised Apart from Alcoholic Biological Parents," *Archives of General Psychiatry*, vol. 28 (1973): 238–243.

9. A. Tolor and J. S. Tamerin, "The Question of a Genetic Basis for Alcoholism: Comment on the Study by Goodwin et al.," *Quarterly Journal of Alcohol Studies*, vol. 34 (1973): 1341–1345.

10. *Alcohol and Health*, second report to U. S. Congress from Department of Health, Education, and Welfare, preprint edition (June, 1974), chap. IV.

11. W. McCord and J. McCord, *Origins of Alcoholism* (Stanford: Stanford University Press, 1960).

12. H. J. Eysenck, *Crime and Personality*, p. 68.

13. A. R. Lindesmith, *Opiate Addiction* (San Antonio, Texas: Principia Press of Trinity University, 1947).

14. Dr. Lee Robins, "A Followup of Vietnam Drug Users," report for U. S. Department of Defense released in press briefing by Richard S. Wilbur, M. D., assistant secretary of defense (April 23, 1973).

15. H. E. Hill, "The Social Deviant and Initial Addiction to Narcotics and Alcohol," *Quarterly Journal of Studies in Alcohol*, vol. 23 (1962): 563.

16. A. Wikler, "A Psychodynamic Study of a Patient During Self-Regulated Re-addiction to Morphine," *Psychiatric Quarterly*, vol. 26 (1952): 270.
  A. Wikler, "Mechanisms of Action of Drugs that Modify Personality Function," *American Journal of Psychiatry*, vol. 108 (1952): 590.

17. E. Preble and J. J. Casey, "Taking Care of Business—The Heroin User's Life on the Street," *International Journal of Addiction*, vol. 4 (1969): 1.

18. *Alcohol and Health*, Second Report to U. S. Congress from Department of Health, Education, and Welfare.

19. F. Anstie, *Stimulants and Narcotics, Their Mutual Relations* (London: Macmillan and Co., 1864).

Chapter 12

1. Ernst Haeckel, *The Wonders of Life*, pp. 118–119.

2. Karl Pearson, *The Scope and Importance to the State of the Science of National Eugenics*, 3rd ed. (London: Dulau, 1911), p. 24.

3. Karl Pearson, "A First Study of the Statistics of Pulmonary Tuberculosis," *Draper's Company Research Memoirs, Studies in National Deterioration*, 2 (London: Dulau, 1907).

4. Emil Rothstein in *Personality, Stress and Tuberculosis* (New York: International Universities Press, 1956).

5. Franz Kallman and D. Reisner, *Journal of Heredity,* vol. 34 (1943): 269 and 293.

   Franz Kallman and D. Reisner, *American Review of Tuberculosis,* vol. 47 (1943): 549.

6. B. Harvald and M. Hauge, *Danish Medical Bulletin,* vol. 3 (1956): 150.

7. Barbara Simonds, *Tuberculosis in Twins* (London: Pitman Publishing Co. Ltd., 1963).

8. John Langdon Down, "Observations on an Ethnic Classification of Idiots," *Clinical Lectures and Reports, London Hospital,* iii (England: 1866), 259–262.

9. Denis Burkitt, "Geographical Pathology Related to Diet," *The Medical Annual* (Bristol: Wright, 1972).

Chapter 13

1. Ida Macalpine and Richard Hunter, *Porphyria: A Royal Malady* (London: British Medical Association, 1968).

2. Ibid.

3. E. Bleuler, *Dementia Praecox or the Group of Schizophrenias* (New York: International Universities Press, 1950).

4. J. E. Cooper et al., *Psychiatric Diagnosis in New York and London,* Institute of Psychiatry Monographs, 20 (London and New York: Oxford University Press, 1972).

5. Dr. Norman Sartorious, *The International Pilot Study of Schizophrenia* (Geneva: WHO, 1973).

6. Thomas S. Szasz, *The Manufacture of Madness* (New York: Harper & Row, 1970; London: Routledge and Kegan Paul, 1971).

7. J. Huxley, E. Mayr, H. Osmond, and A. Hoffer, "Schizophrenia as a Genetic Morphism," *Nature,* vol. 204 (1964): 220.

8. Roland Fischer, "Schizophrenia Research in Biological Perspective," in Arnold R. Kaplan, ed., *Genetic Factors in Schizophrenia* (Springfield, Ill.: Charles C. Thomas, 1972).

9. Professor J. H. Edwards, "The Genetic Basis of Schizophrenia," in Arnold R. Kaplan, ed., *Genetic Factors in Schizophrenia,* p. 310.

10. Seymour S. Kety, David Rosenthal, Paul H. Wender, and Fini Schulsinger, "The Types and Prevalence of Mental Illness in the Biological and Adoptive Families of Adopted Schizophrenics," in David Rosenthal and Seymour S. Kety, eds., *Transmission of Schizophrenia* (New York and London: Pergamon Press, 1968).

Chapter 14

1. H. B. M. Murphy, "The Evocative Role of Complex Tasks," in Arnold R. Kaplan, ed., *Genetic Factors in Schizophrenia.*

2. Ibid.

3. Ibid.

4. H. R. Steinberg and J. Durell, "A Stressful Situation as a Precipitant of Schizophrenic Symptoms," *British Journal of Psychiatry,* vol. 114 (1968): 1097–1105.

5. Gregory Bateson, "Towards a Theory of Schizophrenia," first published with other authors in *Behavioural Science,* vol. 1, no. 4 (1956); reprinted in *Steps to an Ecology of Mind* (London: Paladin, 1973).

6. Ibid.

7. Ibid.

8. Theodore Lidz, "The Family, Language, and the Transmission of Schizophrenia," in David Rosenthal and Seymour S. Kety, eds., *Transmission of Schizophrenia,* p. 180.

9. L. C. Wynne and M. T. Singer, "Thought Disorder and Family Relations of Schizophrenics, II, A Classification of Forms of Thinking," *Archives of General Psychiatry,* vol. 9 (1963): 199–206.

10. L. C. Wynne, "Methodologic and Conceptual Issues in the Study of Schizophrenics and Their Families," in *Transmission of Schizophrenia.*

11. R. D. Laing and A. Esterson, *Sanity, Madness and the Family, vol. 1: Families of Schizophrenics* (London: Tavistock, 1964).

12. R. D. Laing, *The Politics of Experience* (London and Harmondsworth: Penguin, 1967).

13. Donald G. Langsley and David M. Kaplan, *The Treatment of Families in Crisis* (New York and London: Grune and Stratton, 1968).

14. Morton Schatzman, *Soul Murder* (London: Allen Lane, the Penguin Press, 1973).

15. D. P. Schreber, *Dentwürdigkeiten eines Nervenkranken* (Leipzig: Oswald Mutze, 1903), trans. and ed., I. Macalpine and R. A. Hunter: *Memoirs of My Mental Illness* (London: Dawsons of Pall Mall, 1955).

16. D. G. M. Schreber, *Die Schädlichen Korperhaltungen und Gewohnheiten der Kinder nebst Angabe der Mittle Dagegen [The Harmful Body Positions and Habits of Children Including a Statement of Counteracting Measures]* (Leipzig: Fleischer, 1853).

17. D. P. Schreber, *Memoirs of My Mental Illness.*

18. D. G. M. Schreber, *The Harmful Body Positions and Habits of Children.*

19. D. P. Schreber, *Memoirs of My Mental Illness.*

20. Ibid.

21. Ibid.

22. D. G. M. Schreber, *The Harmful Body Positions and Habits of Children.*

23. Ibid.

24. Morton Schatzman, *Soul Murder.*

25. David Rosenthal, *Genetic Theory and Abnormal Behavior* (New York: McGraw-Hill, 1970).

26. H. J. Eysenck and D. B. Prell, "The Inheritance of Neuroticism: An Experimental Study," *Journal of Mental Science,* vol. 97 (1951): 441–467.

27. Duncan Blewett as quoted in J. Shields, "Personality Differences and

Neurotic Traits in Normal Twin School Children," *Eugenics Review,* vol. 45 (1954): 213–246.

28. David Rosenthal, *Genetic Theory and Abnormal Behavior.*

Chapter 15

1. A. Binet, *Les Idées Modernes sur les Enfants* (Paris: Ernest Flamarion, 1909), pp. 54–55. Cited from G. D. Stoddard, "The IQ: Its Ups and Downs," Educational Record, vol. 20 (1939): 44–57.
2. Francis Galton, *Hereditary Genius.*
3. Ibid.
4. L. M. Terman, *The Measurement of Intelligence* (Boston: Houghton Mifflin, 1916).
5. R. M. Yerkes, *Psychological Testing in the U. S. Army* (1921).
6. John Stuart Mill, *Examination of Sir William Hamilton's Philosophy,* chap. 12.
7. J. Helmuth, ed., *Compensatory Education: A National Debate* (New York: Brunner/Mazel, 1970).
8. J. McVicker Hunt, ed., *The Role of Experience in Human Intelligence.*
9. Arthur R. Jensen, "How Much Can We Boost IQ and Scholastic Achievement?"
10. Martin Deutsch, "Happenings on the Way Back to the Forum," *Harvard Educational Review,* vol. 39, no. 3 (Summer, 1969): 525.
11. H. J. Eysenck, *Race, Intelligence and Education.*
12. H. J. Eysenck, *The Inequality of Man* (London: Maurice Temple Smith, 1973).
13. Arthur R. Jensen, "How Much Can We Boost IQ and Scholastic Achievement?"
14. R. C. Lewontin, "Race and Intelligence," *Bulletin of the Atomic Scientists,* vol. 26 (1970): 2–8.
15. Ibid.
16. H. J. Eysenck, *Race, Intelligence and Education.*
17. J. Hirsch, "Behavior-Genetic Analysis and Its Biosocial Consequences," *Seminars in Psychiatry,* vol. 25 (1970): 568.
18. H. J. Eysenck, *Race, Intelligence and Education.*
19. Arthur R. Jensen, "How Much Can We Boost IQ and Scholastic Achievement?"
20. Christopher Jencks et al., *Inequality: A Reassessment of the Effect of Family and Schooling in America* (New York and London: Basic Books Inc., 1972).
21. Arthur R. Jensen, "How Much Can We Boost IQ and Scholastic Achievement?"
22. R. G. Record, T. McKeown, and J. H. Edwards, "An Investigation of the Difference in Measured Intelligence Between Twins and Single Births," *Annals of Human Genetics,* vol. 34 (1970): 11.

23. B. S. Bloom, *Stability and Change in Human Characteristics* (New York: John Wiley, 1964).

24. H. J. Eysenck, *Race, Intelligence and Education.*

25. Walter F. Bodmer and Luigi Luca Cavalli-Sforza, "Intelligence and Race," *Scientific American,* vol. 223 (October, 1970): 19–29.

26. J. M. Thoday, "Educability and Group Differences," *Nature,* vol. 245 (London: October, 1973).

27. Ibid.

Chapter 16

1. William Shockley quoted in "Leeds Snub for Professor," diary story in *The* (London) *Times* (February 15, 1973).

2. William Shockley, "Human Quality Problems and Research Taboos."

3. Ibid.

4. William Shockley, McMaster University Lecture, December, 1967, as quoted by Shockley in letter to Palo Alto *Times* (December 28, 1967).

5. John Howard Griffin, *Black Like Me* (Boston: Houghton Mifflin, 1961; London: Panther Books, 1964).

6. William Shockley, "Moral Obligation to Diagnose the Origin of Negro IQ Deficits," *Review of Educational Research,* vol. 41, no. 4 (1971): 369–377.

7. William Shockley, talk given in spring, 1967, quoted in *Science,* vol. 158 (1967): 892.

8. William Shockley, "Human Quality Problems and Research Taboos."

9. National Academy of Sciences (Washington, D. C.) statement on "Human Genetics and Urban Slums," *Science,* vol. 158 (1967): 892–893.

10. Ibid.

11. William Shockley, "Human Quality Problems and Research Taboos."

Chapter 17

1. H. M. Skeels and H. B. Dye, "A Study of the Effects of Differential Stimulation on Mentally Retarded Children," *Proceedings of the American Association for Mental Defects,* vol. 44 (1939): 114–136.

2. H. M. Skeels, "Adult Status of Children with Contrasting Early Life Experiences: A Follow-up Study," Monographs of the Society for Research into Child Development, vol. 35 (1966): 3.

3. M. Skodak, "Adult Status of Individuals Who Experienced Early Intervention," *Proceedings of the First Congress Association for Scientific Study of Mental Deficiency,* 11–18, B. W. Richards, ed. (Reigate, England: Michael Jackson, 1968).

4. Arthur R. Jensen, "How Much Can We Boost IQ and Scholastic Achievement?"

5. B. Nurcombe, P. de Lacey, Paul Moffit, and Lorne Taylor, "The Question of Aboriginal Intelligence," *The Medical Journal of Australia* (September 29, 1973): 625–635.

6. Rick Heber et al., "Rehabilitation of Families at Risk for Mental Retardation," *Progress Report from Rehabilitation Research Center* (Madison: University of Wisconsin, 1972).

7. George W. Mayeske et al., "A Study of the Nation's Schools," a working paper (Washington, D. C.: U. S. Department of Health, Education, and Welfare, undated).

8. Gordon W. Miller, "Factors in School Achievement and Social Class," *Journal of Educational Psychology*, vol. 61 (1970): 260–269.

9. M. L. Fick, The Educability of the South African Native (Pretoria: South African Council for Educational and Social Research, 1939).

10. H. Gordon, "Mental and Scholastic Tests Among Retarded Children," *Board of Education Pamphlet no. 44* (London: Her Majesty's Stationery Office, 1923).

11. Gustav Jahoda, "A Cross-cultural Perspective in Psychology," *Advancement of Science* (September, 1970): 57–70.

12. W. Dennis, "Performance of Near-Eastern Children on the Draw-a-Man Test," *Child Development*, vol. 28 (1957): 427–430.

13. D. Price-Williams, W. Gordon, and M. Ramirez, "Skill and Conservation," *Developmental Psychology*, vol. 1 (1969): 769.

14. Robert C. Annis and Barrie Frost, "Human Visual Ecology and Orientation Anisotropies in Acuity," *Science*, 16 (November, 1973): 729–731.

Chapter 18

1. Richard Herrnstein, *I.Q. in the Meritocracy*.

2. Liam Hudson, "Selection and the Problem of Conformity," *Genetic and Environmental Factors in Human Ability*, ed. J. E. Meade and A. S. Parkes (Edinburgh: Oliver and Boyd, 1966).

3. D. W. Mackinnon, "The Nature and Nurture of Creative Talent," *American Psychologist*, vol. 17 (1962): 484.

4. A. Anastasi, "Intelligence and Family Size," *Psychological Bulletin*, vol. 53 (1956): 187–209.

5. J. E. Meade, "Inheritance of Inequalities," lecture delivered to the British Academy (December, 1973).

6. David Boyd, *Elites and Their Education* (London: National Foundation for Educational Research, 1973).

Chapter 19

1. Jacques Barzun, *Race: A Study in Superstition* (first published in 1937, revised as Harper Torchbook edition, 1965).

2. H. J. Eysenck, *Race, Intelligence and Education*.

3. H. J. Muller, *Out of the Night: A Biologist's View of the Future* (New York: Vanguard, 1935).

4. H. J. Muller, "The Guidance of Human Evolution," *Perspectives in Biology and Medicine*, vol. 3 (1959): 1–43; also in S. Tax, *Evolution After Darwin*: 423–462.

5. Judge Gerhardt A. Gesell, judgment in action concerning the Relf sisters,

quoted in *New England Journal of Medicine,* "Law-Medicine Notes" (see below).

6. William J. Curran, J. D. "Sterilization of the Poor: Judge Gesell's Road-block," in "Law-Medicine Notes," *The New England Journal of Medicine,* vol. 291 (July, 1974): 25–26.

7. "Sterilization Guidelines: 22 Months on the Shelf," *Medical World News* (November 9, 1973); "HEW Sterilization Rules Blasted" (September 7, 1973).

8. J. W. Olney and L. G. Sharpe, "Brain Lesions in Infant Monkeys Treated with Sodium Glutamate," *Science,* vol. 166 (1969): 386–388; J. W. Olney, L. G. Sharpe, and R. D. Feigin, "Glutamate-Induced Brain Damage in Infant Primates," *Journal of Neuropathology and Experimental Neurology,* vol. 31: 464–488.

Index

vaginal transplants, 61-62
Valium, 138
Vavilov, 26
Verschuer, Otto von, 30-31, 142
Victoria, Queen, 21
Vinci, Leonardo da, 78

Wade, Nicholas, 118
Wagner, Gerhardt, 93
Walzer, Stanley, 121-122
Ward, Ingelborg, 75
Warhol, Andy, 86
Watson, James, 20
Watson, John B., 45
Well of Loneliness, The, 80
Wender, Paul, 158
West, D. J., 87
Whatmore, P. B., 116-117
Whitman, Walt, 78
Widdowson, Elsie M., 125

Wikler, Abraham, 137
Wilde, Oscar, 78
Wilson, Albert, 115
woman's liberation movement, 51
women:
  domesticity of, 91, 93, 94, 95, 96-97,
    163-164
  fear of success in, 90, 91-92, 96
  heredity and position of, 51
  mental illness in, 163-164, 165-166
World War II, stress in, 164-165
Wyndham, Francis, 109
Wynne, Lyman, 167, 168

X and Y chromosomes, *see* chromosomes

Y-factor criminal, 99, 115-123
Yerkes, R. M., 181